DR. JOHN CAMBRIDGE PHD

Overweight treatment

Contents

1.

2.

3.

4.

5.

6.

7.

8.

9.

10.

11.

12.

13.

14.

INTRODUCTION.

The groundbreaking book The Overweight treatment explores the reasons for the obesity epidemic's underlying problems and offers sustainable remedies. It uses data from countless scientific studies, journals, and meta-analyses that span decades of research. To achieve the ideal body composition and metabolic health, it is essential to educate people about the factors that contribute to overweight treatment and weight increase. The overweight treatment aims to teach you how to become the master of your body and fat reduction rather than recommending any certain diet or banning others.

CHAPTER 1: Always Eat Balanced Meals.

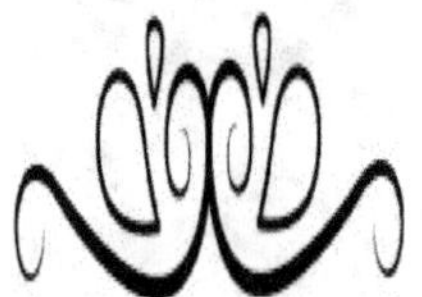

Always Eat Balanced Meals.

Eating balanced meals plays a crucial role in maintaining good health and well-being. It involves consuming a variety of foods from different food groups in appropriate portions to ensure that the body receives all the essential nutrients it needs to function optimally. In this article, we will delve into the importance of balanced eating, the key components of a balanced meal, and some practical tips for incorporating balance into your daily diet.

A balanced meal consists of macronutrients (carbohydrates, proteins, and fats) along with micronutrients (vitamins and minerals) in the right proportions. These nutrients have specific roles in the body, and their adequate intake is vital for maintaining energy levels, supporting growth and repair, boosting immunity, and promoting overall well-being.

Carbohydrates are the primary source of energy and are found in foods like grains, cereals, fruits, and vegetables. They provide glucose, which fuels our brain and muscles. Including complex carbohydrates like whole grains and fiber-rich foods helps in maintaining steady blood sugar levels and provides sustained energy throughout the day.

Proteins are essential for building and repairing tissues, producing enzymes and hormones, and maintaining a healthy immune system. Good sources of protein include lean meats, poultry, fish, dairy products, legumes, and plant-based options like tofu and tempeh. It is important to consume a variety of protein sources to ensure the intake of all essential amino acids.

Fats are vital for hormone production, insulation of organs, absorption of fat-soluble vitamins, and providing an additional source of energy. Opt for healthier fats like unsaturated fats found in nuts, seeds, avocados, and olive oil while limiting saturated and trans fats found in fried foods and processed snacks.

Micronutrients, such as vitamins and minerals, are required in smaller quantities but are equally important. They support various bodily functions, including maintaining strong bones, boosting immunity, and aiding in the production of red blood cells. Include a variety of fruits, vegetables, nuts, seeds, whole grains, and lean proteins to ensure a diverse array of micronutrient intake.

Now that we understand the components of a balanced meal, let's discuss why it is essential to always eat balanced meals:

1. **Optimal nutrient intake:** Consuming a balanced meal ensures that the body receives all the necessary nutrients in adequate amounts. This helps prevent deficiencies and ensures optimal functioning of the body's systems.

2. **Boosts energy levels:** Balanced meals provide a steady supply of energy throughout the day, avoiding energy dips and maintaining optimal productivity and mental focus.

3. **Weight management:** Balanced meals help regulate appetite and prevent overeating. Including a combination of carbohydrates, proteins, and fats promotes satiety, reducing the likelihood of snacking on unhealthy, calorie-dense foods.

4. **Supports overall health:** A balanced diet aids in maintaining a healthy weight, reducing the risk of chronic diseases like obesity, heart disease, diabetes, and certain types of cancer. It also supports digestive health, prevents nutrient deficiencies, and strengthens the immune system.

incorporation rate balanced eating into your daily routine, consider the following tips:

1. **Plan your meals:** Take some time to plan your meals and snacks in advance. This allows you to ensure a variety of foods from different food groups are included in your diet.

2. **Portion control:** Pay attention to your portion sizes. Use smaller plates and bowls to avoid overeating, and aim to fill half of your plate with colorful fruits and vegetables, one-

quarter with lean proteins, and one-quarter with whole grains or other complex carbohydrates.

3. **Incorporate variety:** Don't stick to the same foods every day. Experiment with different fruits, vegetables, grains, and proteins to keep your meals interesting and ensure a wide range of nutrients.

4. **Practice moderation:** While it is important to eat a balanced diet, it is also essential to enjoy your favorite treats in moderation. Depriving yourself of occasional indulgences may make it more challenging to stick to a balanced eating plan in the long run.

5. **Stay hydrated:** Water is vital for overall health. Drink plenty of water throughout the day to stay hydrated and support optimal bodily functions.

To wrap up, always prioritizing balanced meals is essential for maintaining good health and well-being. By including a variety of macronutrients and micronutrients in appropriate proportions, you can support your body's needs and enjoy the benefits of sustained energy, improved focus, weight management, and overall health. So remember, make balanced eating a fundamental part of your lifestyle for a happier, healthier you.

Maintaining a balanced diet is essential for overall health and well-being. It involves consuming a variety of nutrients in appropriate proportions to ensure you meet your body's nutritional requirements. In this summary, we will explore the importance of always eating balanced meals by providing tips, causes, factors, benefits, advantages, and disadvantages.

Tips for Always Eating Balanced Meals:

1. **Plan your meals:** Taking the time to plan your meals in advance helps ensure that you include a variety of nutritious foods in your diet.

2. **Include all food groups:** A balanced meal consists of carbohydrates, proteins, healthy fats, vitamins, and minerals. Incorporate diverse foods from each food group into your meals.

3. **Portion control:** Be mindful of portion sizes and avoid overeating. Use smaller plates to help control portion sizes.

4. **Prioritize whole foods:** Opt for whole grains, lean proteins, fruits, vegetables, and healthy fats rather than processed and refined foods.

5. **Limit sugary beverages:** High sugar content in beverages can lead to weight gain and other health issues. Choose water, herbal teas, or natural fruit juices instead.

6. **Snack smartly:** Choose healthy snacks like nuts, seeds, fruits, or yogurt instead of reaching for processed snacks high in unhealthy fats and sugars.

7. **Cook at home:** Preparing homemade meals gives you control over the ingredients, helping avoid excessive sodium, unhealthy fats, and added sugars commonly found in restaurant or packaged meals.

8. **Read food labels:** Be aware of hidden ingredients, such as excessive salt, sugar, or unhealthy fats in processed foods. Reading labels can help you make informed choices.

9. **Practice mindful eating:** Pay attention to your body's hunger and fullness cues. Eat slowly, savor each bite, and listen to your body's signals to prevent overeating.

10. **Seek professional advice:** Consult a registered dietitian or nutritionist to create a personalized meal plan if you have specific dietary needs or health concerns.

Causes of Nutritional Imbalance:

1. **Poor food choices:** Frequent consumption of processed and fast foods can lead to an unbalanced diet lacking essential nutrients.

2. **Busy lifestyles:** Time constraints may lead to reliance on convenience foods that often lack nutritional value.

3. **Emotional eating:** Using food as a coping mechanism can result in imbalanced food choices and nutrient deficiencies.

4. **Lack of knowledge:** Many individuals may lack the necessary knowledge about nutrition, which can contribute to unbalanced diets.

5. **Food deserts:** Living in areas with limited access to fresh and healthy foods can make it challenging to maintain a balanced diet.

6. **Inadequate cooking skills:** Difficulty in preparing nutritious meals can lead to an imbalance in food choices.

7. **Financial constraints:** Limited budgets may result in purchasing cheaper, less nutritious food options.

8. **Dietary restrictions or allergies:** Certain dietary restrictions or allergies can limit food choices, potentially leading to nutritional imbalances.

9. **Disrupted eating patterns:** Skipping meals or irregular eating habits can lead to inadequate nutrient intake.

10. **Lack of parental guidance:** Insufficient guidance from parents or caregivers in early life may result in unhealthy eating habits that persist into adulthood.

Factors Influencing Balanced Eating:

1. **Age and gender:** Nutritional requirements vary based on age and gender, with different needs during growth, pregnancy, and lactation.

2. **Metabolic rate:** Individual metabolic rates affect calorie needs and nutrient requirements. Some individuals may require higher or lower intake to maintain energy balance.

3. **Physical activity level:** Active individuals have higher energy requirements and may need increased protein and nutrient intake to support muscle recovery and growth.

4. **Health conditions:** Certain health conditions require specific dietary modifications to manage symptoms or support treatment.

5. **Mental health:** Emotional well-being can influence eating behaviors and food choices. Individuals experiencing mental health issues may struggle with maintaining balanced diets.

6. **Cultural and religious beliefs:** Cultural and religious practices can influence food choices and dietary restrictions.

7. **Socioeconomic status:** Economic factors may impact access to nutritious foods, affecting the ability to maintain balanced diets.

8. **Environmental factors:** Availability of fresh produce, local food culture, and advertising practices shape dietary patterns in different regions.

9. **Peer and social influence:** Social factors can influence food choices, often leading to unhealthy dietary habits.

10. **Education:** Knowledge about nutrition and understanding how to create balanced meals plays a crucial role in promoting healthy eating habits.

Benefits of Following a Balanced Diet:

1. **Optimal nutrient intake:** Consuming a balanced diet ensures sufficient intake of essential nutrients for overall health and well-being.

2. **Weight management:** A balanced diet, combined with regular physical activity, can help maintain a healthy weight and prevent obesity.

3. **Enhanced energy levels:** Proper nutrient intake fuels the body, providing energy for physical and mental activities.

4. **Improved digestion:** A balanced diet rich in fiber promotes healthy digestion and prevents digestive issues like constipation.

5. **Strong immune system:** Balanced meals provide vital vitamins and minerals, supporting a robust immune system and reducing the risk of infections.

6. **Reduced risk of chronic diseases:** A balanced diet lowers the risk of conditions like heart disease, diabetes, certain cancers, and hypertension.

7. **Mental well-being:** Nutrient-dense foods contribute to improved cognitive function and mental well-being.

8. **Healthy skin and hair:** A balanced diet rich in essential fatty acids, vitamins, and minerals promotes healthy skin and hair.

9. **Better sleep quality:** A nutritious diet positively influences sleep patterns, promoting restful sleep and overall well-being.

10. **Longevity:** Following a balanced diet promotes a healthier lifestyle, increasing the chances of living a longer, disease-free life.

Advantages of Always Eating Balanced Meals:

1. **Enhanced overall health:** Consistently consuming balanced meals leads to improved overall health, preventing nutrient deficiencies and associated health issues.

2. **Stable energy levels:** Balanced meals provide a steady supply of energy throughout the day, reducing energy slumps.

3. **Increased productivity:** Proper nutrition fuels cognitive function, increasing productivity levels and focus.

4. **Optimal physical performance:** Adequate nutrient intake supports physical performance, endurance, and recovery in athletes and active individuals.

5. **Maintenance of healthy weight:** Eating balanced meals helps manage weight by promoting portion control and providing essential nutrients.

6. **Reduced risk of chronic diseases:** A balanced diet lowers the risk of chronic diseases like heart disease, diabetes, and certain cancers.

7. **Improved digestion and gut health:** A diet rich in fiber and nutrients promotes a healthy digestive system and gut microbiome.

8. **Strengthened immune system:** Balanced meals supply essential vitamins, minerals, and antioxidants, boosting the immune system.

9. **Enhanced mood and mental well-being:** Nutrient-dense foods support brain health, positively impacting mood and overall mental well-being.

10. **Long-term sustainability:** Adopting a balanced eating habit ensures long-term sustainability and promotes a healthier lifestyle for a lifetime.

Disadvantages of Ignoring Balanced Eating:

1. **Nutrient deficiencies:** Ignoring balanced eating can lead to nutrient deficiencies, causing various health issues like anemia, osteoporosis, or weakened immune function.

2. **Weight gain or obesity:** An unbalanced diet high in calories, unhealthy fats, and sugars increases the risk of weight gain and obesity.

3. **Lack of energy and fatigue:** Poor nutrition can result in low energy levels and chronic fatigue.

4. **Increased risk of chronic diseases:** A diet lacking essential nutrients increases the risk of developing chronic diseases like heart disease, diabetes, or certain cancers.

5. **Poor digestion and gut health:** Insufficient fiber and nutrients can result in digestive problems like constipation, bloating, or an imbalanced gut microbiome.

6. **Impaired cognitive function:** Inadequate nutrition negatively impacts cognitive abilities, memory, and focus.

7. **Weakened immune system:** A lack of essential vitamins and minerals weakens the immune system, making the body more susceptible to infections and illnesses.

8. **Skin and hair issues:** Poor nutrition reflects on the skin and hair, leading to issues like acne, dryness, or brittle hair.

9. **Increased mood fluctuations:** Imbalanced eating patterns can contribute to mood swings, irritability, and mental health concerns.

10. **Reduced quality of life:** Ignoring balanced eating negatively affects overall health and well-being, reducing the quality of life in the long run.

In conclusion, always eating balanced meals offers numerous benefits for physical and mental health. By following the ten tips mentioned, understanding the causes and factors that influence balanced eating, and being mindful of the associated benefits and advantages, individuals can make informed choices and work towards maintaining a balanced diet. Ignoring this essential aspect of nutrition may result in nutrient deficiencies, chronic diseases, and a reduced overall quality of life. Therefore, it is crucial to prioritize balanced eating for optimal health and well-being.

CHAPTER 2: Foods High In Fat But Don't Make You Fat.

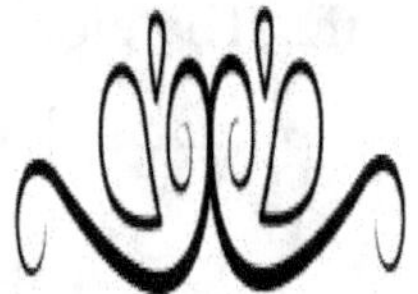

Foods High In Fat But Don't Make You Fat.

Foods high in fat have long been associated with weight gain and negative health effects. However, not all high-fat foods contribute to weight gain. In fact, there are several foods that are high in fat but don't necessarily make you fat. This article will provide a summary of foods that are high in fat but can still be part of a healthy diet and may even have certain health benefits.

Firstly, it's important to understand that not all fats are created equal. There are different types of fats, including saturated fats, unsaturated fats, and trans fats. Saturated fats, found in animal products like meat and dairy, as well as some plant-based oils like coconut oil, have been associated with an increased risk of heart disease when consumed in excess. Trans fats, found in processed foods like fried and baked goods, are also considered harmful to health.

On the other hand, unsaturated fats, which can be further categorized into monounsaturated fats and polyunsaturated fats, are considered healthier fats. These fats are found in foods like avocados, nuts, seeds, and fatty fish like salmon. They provide essential fatty acids and have been associated with various health benefits, including improved heart health, reduced inflammation, and better brain function.

One reason why foods high in fat don't necessarily make you fat is that fat is a highly satiating macronutrient. When consumed in reasonable amounts, fat can help you feel fuller for longer, reducing the overall calorie intake. This can be particularly beneficial for weight management as it can help control appetite and prevent overeating.

Moreover, certain high-fat foods are nutrient-dense and provide a range of important vitamins and minerals. For example, avocados are high in monounsaturated fats and are also a good source of fiber, potassium, vitamin K, vitamin E, and vitamin C. Nuts and seeds are rich in healthy fats, as well as protein, fiber, and various micronutrients like vitamin E, magnesium, and zinc. Including these foods in a balanced diet can contribute to overall nutrient intake and support overall health.

Another aspect to consider is the role of fat in nutrient absorption. Some vitamins, such as vitamins A, D, E, and K, are fat-soluble, meaning they require fat for optimal absorption. Including healthy fats in meals that contain these vitamins can enhance their absorption and utilization by the body.

Furthermore, research has shown that certain high-fat foods can have metabolic benefits. For example, extra virgin olive oil, which is high in monounsaturated fats, has been associated with reduced inflammation, improved heart health, and a lower risk of chronic diseases like type 2 diabetes and certain types of cancer. Fatty fish, such as salmon, mackerel, and sardines, are high in omega-3 fatty acids, which have anti-inflammatory properties and are crucial for brain health.

It's important to note that while some high-fat foods can be part of a healthy diet, portion control and overall calorie intake still play a significant role in weight management. Consuming excess calories, regardless of the macronutrient composition, can lead to weight gain. Therefore, it's important to consume high-fat foods in moderation as part of a balanced diet that includes a variety of nutrient-rich foods.

In summary, not all high-fat foods contribute to weight gain or negative health effects. Healthy fats, such as those found in avocados, nuts, seeds, and fatty fish, can be part of a balanced diet and provide various health benefits. These foods can help increase satiety, provide essential nutrients, support nutrient absorption, and even have metabolic benefits. However, portion control and overall calorie intake are still important factors to consider for weight management. Incorporating a variety of nutrient-rich foods, including foods high in healthy fats, can contribute to a well-rounded and healthy diet.

Foods high in fat can still be incorporated into a balanced diet without causing weight gain. Here are some tips, causes, functions, advantages, and disadvantages of such foods.

Tips:

1. **Moderation:** Enjoy high-fat foods in moderation to maintain a healthy balance with other nutrients.
2. **Choose healthy fats:** Opt for foods high in healthy fats, such as avocado, nuts, and olive oil, over saturated and trans fats.
3. **Portion control:** Be mindful of portion sizes when consuming high-fat foods to avoid overeating.
4. **Pair with whole foods:** Combine high-fat foods with fiber-rich options like fruits, vegetables, and whole grains for a more balanced meal.
5. **Mindful cooking methods:** Cook with minimal added fats or use healthier cooking techniques like roasting or grilling.
6. **Read labels:** Check food labels for hidden sources of unhealthy fats or added sugars.
7. **Stay active:** Engage in regular physical activity to burn calories and maintain a healthy weight.
8. **Balanced diet:** Ensure that your overall diet includes a variety of nutrient-rich foods beyond just high-fat options.
9. **Hydration:** Stay hydrated by consuming sufficient water alongside high-fat foods to aid digestion.

10. **Seek professional advice:** Consult a registered dietitian or nutritionist for personalized guidance on incorporating high-fat foods into your diet.

Causes:

1. **Genetic factors:** Some individuals have genes that affect their metabolism of fats, making them less likely to gain weight from fat consumption.
2. **Hormonal influences:** Hormones like leptin and ghrelin can affect appetite regulation and metabolism, influencing how fats are utilized in the body.
3. **Thermic effect:** High-fat foods have a higher thermic effect, which means they require more energy to digest, leading to a slight increase in calorie expenditure.
4. **Exercise level:** Regular physical activity can help increase the body's metabolic rate, allowing for better fat utilization.
5. **Metabolic rate:** Individuals with a naturally higher metabolic rate may process fats more efficiently, reducing the likelihood of weight gain.
6. **Nutrient partitioning:** The body's ability to partition nutrients determines whether fats are stored as fat or utilized for energy.
7. **Gut microbiota:** The composition of gut bacteria can influence the body's ability to digest and utilize fats effectively.

8. **Meal timing:** Consuming high-fat foods at specific times, such as post-workout, can aid in nutrient absorption and utilization.
9. **Emotional eating:** Emotional triggers can lead to overeating, irrespective of the type of food consumed, including high-fat options.
10. **Overall energy balance:** The total amount of calories consumed versus expended throughout the day plays a crucial role in weight management.

Functions:

1. **Energy source:** Fats provide a concentrated form of energy, with 1 gram containing 9 calories, making them an efficient fuel source for the body.
2. **Nutrient absorption:** Some essential vitamins, such as vitamins A, D, E, and K, require fat for proper absorption in the body.
3. **Satiety:** Including healthy fats in your meals can help promote feelings of fullness and reduce the likelihood of overeating.
4. **Insulation:** Fat acts as an insulating layer, protecting vital organs and regulating body temperature.
5. **Cell function:** Fats are important for the structure and function of cell membranes in the body.
6. **Hormonal production:** Fat is crucial for the production of hormones, including sex hormones and certain metabolic hormones.

7. **Brain health:** Essential fatty acids, like omega-3 and omega-6, are important for brain development, cognition, and overall brain health.
8. **Taste and texture:** Fats enhance the taste, texture, and mouthfeel of food, making meals more enjoyable.
9. **Nerve function:** Fatty acids play a role in the transmission of nerve impulses throughout the body.
10. **Flavor carrier:** Fats can carry and enhance the flavors of other ingredients in recipes, adding depth to dishes.

Advantages:

1. **Enhanced satiety:** High-fat foods can keep you feeling fuller for longer, reducing the tendency to overeat.
2. **Improved taste:** Fats add richness and flavor to dishes, making them more enjoyable.
3. **Nutrient absorption:** Fat-soluble vitamins require dietary fat for proper absorption and utilization.
4. **Energy-dense:** Fats provide a concentrated source of energy, beneficial for individuals with high energy requirements, such as athletes.
5. **Essential fatty acids:** Some fats contain essential fatty acids that the body cannot produce on its own but needs for various physiological functions.
6. **Hormone regulation:** Healthy fats play a role in hormone production and regulation, affecting various bodily processes.
7. **Brain health:** Certain fats, like omega-3 fatty acids, support brain health and cognitive function.

8. **Skin and hair health:** Healthy fats contribute to maintaining healthy skin and promoting shiny hair.

9. **Flavor enhancement:** Fats can enhance the taste and mouthfeel of various foods.

10. **Long-term sustainability:** Including moderate amounts of healthy fats in the diet can contribute to a sustainable, enjoyable, and balanced eating pattern.

Disadvantages:

1. **High calorie content:** Fats are calorie-dense, and excessive consumption can lead to weight gain if not balanced with overall energy intake.

2. **Unhealthy fats:** Some high-fat foods are also high in unhealthy saturated and trans fats, which can be detrimental to heart health when consumed in excess.

3. **Portion control challenges:** Overconsumption of high-fat foods can be a challenge when it comes to portion control due to their palatability.

4. **Lack of nutrient diversity:** Relying heavily on high-fat foods may limit the intake of other essential nutrients from a diverse range of food sources.

5. **Saturation point:** The body has a limited capacity to digest and utilize fats efficiently, leading to potential storage if consumed in excess.

6. **Nutrient imbalance:** Focusing solely on high-fat foods may result in an imbalance in other macronutrients like protein and carbohydrates.

7. **Digestive issues:** Some individuals may experience digestive discomfort, such as bloating or diarrhea, when consuming high-fat foods, especially in large amounts.
8. **Heart health concerns:** A diet high in unhealthy fats can increase the risk of heart disease, high cholesterol, and other cardiovascular issues.
9. **Weight management challenges:** While high-fat foods may not directly cause weight gain, excessive consumption can still contribute to an unhealthy overall energy balance.
10. Individual variations: Each person's response to high-fat foods can differ based on factors like genetics, metabolism, and overall lifestyle, making it important to monitor individual health markers and seek personalized advice.

Please note that consultation with a qualified healthcare professional or registered dietitian is always recommended to determine an appropriate diet based on individual needs and health concerns.

Foods High In Fat But Don't Make You Fat.

You are not your food. People who consume a lot of fat would be obese if we were what we ate. Your body requires dietary fat to function effectively and lose weight, which is why many fats are referred to as "essential." Healthy fats promote your body's absorption of fat-soluble vitamins, control hunger hormones, increase satiety, guard against heart disease, and carry nutrients through your body. Not to mention that many of those essential elements, including vitamins, minerals, and antioxidants that combat free radicals, are bundled with the majority of unprocessed, high-fat foods. We identified the top foods with healthy fats so you can add them to your diet with ease. But first, hold on On a high-fat binge, keep in mind that even these good fats should be eaten in proportion, just like all other foods.

1. Grass-fed beef.

Conjugated linoleic acid, or CLA, the trans fat that helps reduce belly fat and enhance heart health, and stearic acid, a saturated fat that lowers LDL cholesterol are two of the good fats that come from red meat. However, grass-fed beef is superior to the variety you usually choose. A study published in the Nutrition Journal found that grass-fed beef has lower levels of unhealthy palmitic acid than beef that has been raised conventionally and is higher in CLA, stearic acid, and omega-3 fatty acids (because grass contains ALA and corn does not). Grass-fed beef is also naturally leaner and contains fewer calories than conventional meat, which is good news for your waistline.

2. Coconut.

The saturated fat content of coconut is considerable, but more than half of that is made up of lauric acid, a special medium-chain triglyceride that fights germs, lowers cholesterol, and, according to a Journal of Nutrition research, can raise a person's 24-hour energy expenditure by as much as 5%. What's more? According to a study in the journal Lipids, adding coconut oil to one's diet can truly help reduce belly fat. To start trimming your waist, top yogurt with unsweetened flakes and stir-fry with coconut oil.

3. Avocado.

Avocados are at the forefront of the good fat brigade. This amazing fruit is the butter of nature. It is creamy and delicious, and unlike butter, it is a meal in and of itself. Although you should still keep it to You don't need to be afraid of avocado's fats if you eat a quarter or half of one every meal. According to a Food Function study, avocados contain oleic acid, a healthy monounsaturated lipid that can aid reduce sensations of hunger. Additionally, they provide you with fiber and protein, which butter does not.

4. Chocolate, dark.

Good news, chocolate lovers! Dark chocolate specifically can aid with tummy reduction. Dark chocolate has the largest concentration of pure cocoa butter, which is a source of stearic acid, a saturated fat that slows digestion. Dark chocolate curbs hunger and aids in weight loss since it takes longer to metabolize. In addition to the beneficial lipids, dark chocolate is a rich source of antioxidants, including polyphenols and flavonoids like epicatechin, catechin, and Especially procyanidins, which might enhance blood flow to the brain and fight off free radicals (perhaps making you smarter!). You only need a few ounces of dark chocolate each day to get the advantages.

5. Nuts.

Get crazy! Nuts' polyunsaturated fats trigger genes that lower fat synthesis and enhance insulin metabolism. One of the best dietary sources is walnuts, which contain about 13 grams per one-ounce serving. We discovered that consuming a lot of walnuts and walnut oil may improve how well the body handles stress and lower diastolic blood pressure. Not only that, but a study published in the International Journal Of Obesity and Related Even when two groups of volunteers ingested the same number of calories, Metabolic Disorders discovered that the group that got more calories from fatty almonds lost the most weight. In the end, all nuts will be excellent suppliers of monounsaturated, polyunsaturated, and omega-3 fatty acids, but in different proportions.

6. Nut Butter.

Nut kinds of butter and nuts are similar in many ways, but you might be shocked to learn that not all nut kinds of butter are rich sources of healthful fats. The nutrition information on jars of conventional and reduced-fat nut kinds of butter should be carefully read. You'll notice a few variations: Surprisingly, reduced-fat kinds of butter contain less fat, but they also contain more sugar and salt. Not ideal when trading beneficial monounsaturated fats lipids that aid in reducing your sensitivity to insulin for sugars that raise insulin levels. Make careful to keep things simple and natural. Partially hydrogenated oils, a type of harmful trans fat, can be found in nut kinds of butter that are not natural.

7. Whole eggs.

Not the shells; the yolks. If you're among those who are still unsure about whether you should eat the yolk, the answer is yes! There is no reason to fear, even if the yolk contains fat and cholesterol and the whites are entirely composed of protein. Since most of the fat in egg yolks is monounsaturated, eating more of it will ultimately help lower LDL ("bad" cholesterol). In addition to lowering your cholesterol, eggs are the top dietary source of the nutrient choline. Choline, which can also be found in The gene process that causes your body to retain fat around your liver is attacked by lean meats, shellfish, and collard greens.

8. Greek yogurt.

Yogurt is one of the healthiest foods you can eat for weight loss and overall health because it is loaded with protein, calcium, and probiotics. Make sure you choose Greek, though. Greek yogurt made from whole milk often contains more protein, fat, and less sugar than its leaner counterparts, which provides for the ideal hunger-suppressing combination: because protein takes longer to break down than fat, you won't feel the need for a snack as you go about your morning. Yogurt contains monounsaturated, polyunsaturated, and naturally occurring trans fats in addition to saturated fats, which make up the majority of its fat-content acids. Since both LDL and HDL are increased, the overall fatty acid profile is rather balanced, therefore it won't have a significant impact on cholesterol levels.

9. Salmon, wild.

Salmon may not have the same negative reputation for being high in fat, but its health advantages are still important to note. You may consume the full amount of heart-healthy omega-3 fatty acids advised by the American Heart Association by including this fish fillet in your diet just twice a week. Omega-3 fatty acids lower triglyceride levels, lower blood pressure, and diminish the risk of arrhythmia. Make sure to choose the right fish when you're at the fish counter; farmed Atlantic salmon is the best fish for nutrition and health benefits, while pink salmon is the second-best among the worst.

10. Olive Oil.

This olive oil from the Mediterranean region is high in oleic acid, a monounsaturated fatty acid that strengthens the heart and fights cancer. An olive oil-rich diet produced higher levels of adiponectin than did a high-carb or high-protein diet, supporting the idea that this fat can help you get thin. Adiponectin is a hormone that aids in the breakdown of body fat; hence, the more of it you have, the lower your BMI tends to be. Extra virgin olive oil may raise blood levels of serotonin, a hormone linked to satiety, another reason why you should use this lipid in your sauces and dressings.

11. Heavy Cream and Milk.

Get fat? Full-fat dairy is more filling even though it contains more calories. people who consume fatty foods compared to people who strive to cut calories and fat by eating low-fat dairy are less likely to be obese. Furthermore, neither heart disease nor diabetes was linked to full-fat dairy, according to the study's authors. Ironically, some milk fat acids—those you can't receive from zero-fat varieties—might stimulate your body's calorie-burning organs. Therefore, add heavy cream to your next cup of coffee. According to nutritionist Cassie Bjork, RD, LD, "Heavy cream is a healthy fat that helps keep your blood sugar constant between meals and snacks, which means consistent energy and brain power—not to mention it makes your coffee taste luscious!"

12. Canola Oil.

The broccoli family plant whose seeds are used to make canola oil has a nearly ideal 2.5:1 omega-6 to omega-3 ratio of fats. People who obtain a diet with a ratio like this have reportedly had better success fighting cancer, arthritis, and asthma, according to a study review that was published in Experimental Biology and Medicine. Alpha-linolenic acid (ALA), an important omega-3 fatty acid that may aid in weight maintenance, is also abundant in neutral oil.

13. Tuna.

One of the top suppliers of the omega-3 fatty acid docosahexaenoic acid (DHA) among all the fish in the ocean is tuna. One of the best and most economical fish for weight loss, especially from your belly, is canned light tuna. A study published in the Journal of Lipid Research demonstrated that taking supplements of omega-3 fatty acids had a significant impact on turning off genes for abdominal fat. While DHA and eicosapentaenoic acid (EPA), two types of fatty acids found in cold water fish and fish oils, can be 40 to 70 percent more efficient than EPA at controlling fat genes in the abdomen and limiting the growth of belly fat cells, according to study.

14. Cheese.

Cheese is a great source of protein, calcium, vitamins, minerals, and fatty acids. It also aids in the slowing down of sugar and carbohydrate absorption, resulting in a steady supply of energy and enhanced cognitive function. People who consume a lot of high-fat dairy products have the lowest incidence of diabetes, while those who consume a lot of low-fat dairy products have the highest incidence. This may also help lower your risk of developing diabetes. The Researchers hypothesized that although cheese contains beneficial elements like calcium, protein, vitamin D, and others, humans need fat to benefit from these nutrients' protective properties. Just be certain that it is genuine, full-fat cheese and not wood chips.

15. Flax and chia seeds.

A vital omega-3 fatty acid found in flax and chia seeds, ALA, can help with weight management and may lower the risk of heart disease by improving blood vessel function and lowering inflammation. Omega-3 fatty acids have been shown to increase fat burning and reduce appetite, according to a recent review in the journal Nutrients, and they also boost our body's ability to metabolize fat when consumed in appropriate amounts by changing the way some "fat genes" work.

16. Duck.

Duck contains the largest concentration of arachidonic acid (AA), a type of polyunsaturated fat that helps build muscle, among any lean meats. Men's anaerobic power, strength, and lean body mass have all been found to increase with arachidonic acid supplementation. Men who took AA acquired 3.4 pounds more lean muscle mass than those who took a placebo in a University of Tampa research. By consuming these foods, you may keep upping the burn and get a toned body.

17. Spirulina.

This powdered and supplemented blue-green alga is rich in beneficial omega-3 fatty acids like EPA and DHA. According to research, these types of omega-3s are more effective than ALA at reducing inflammation in the body and abdominal fat Spirulina is not only a fantastic source of heart-healthy lipids, but it's also incredibly high in protein, a fantastic source of probiotics, and it might even be able to help you flatten your stomach while working out. In a study published in Medicine & Science in Sports & Exercise, nine moderately active males took either spirulina capsules or a placebo for four weeks. Those who had taken spirulina pills were able to run 30% longer and burnt 11% more fat during a run than men who had taken a placebo.

18. Bacon.

You read correctly. Even bacon contains good fats! We advise choosing traditional, full-fat pork. While choosing turkey bacon will result in a savings of roughly 13 calories and a gram of fat It also increases the amount of sodium on your plate for each slice, which can cause high blood pressure. Additionally, compared to poultry, the pig provides more protein and heart-healthy monounsaturated fatty acids (MUFAs). No matter what you choose to include on your breakfast plate, keep in mind that portion size is important. All you need   are   a   few   slices.

CHAPTER 3: Causes of Overweight in Foods.

Obesity is a complex health issue influenced by a variety of factors, including genetics, lifestyle, and environmental factors, including diet. In this summary, I will focus on the dietary factors that contribute to obesity.

1. **High-calorie and low-nutrient foods:** Consumption of energy-dense foods that are low in essential nutrients, such as sugary beverages, fast food, processed snacks, and desserts, is strongly associated with weight gain and obesity. These foods often have a high content of added sugars, unhealthy fats, and refined grains, which provide little satiety and can lead to overeating.

2. **Portion sizes:** Oversized portions have become increasingly common, both in restaurants and at home. Larger portion sizes contribute to excessive calorie intake, as people tend to consume more when presented with larger servings. This can lead to weight gain and obesity over time.

3. **Fast food and convenience foods:** The rise of fast food and convenience foods has made it easier for people to access energy-dense, nutrient-poor options. These foods are often high in unhealthy fats, added sugars, and salt, and are typically served in larger portions. Regular consumption of fast food has been linked to weight gain and increased risk of obesity.

4. **Sugar-sweetened beverages:** Sugary beverages, including soda, fruit juices, energy drinks, and sweetened tea and coffee, are a significant contributor to obesity. These drinks are high in added sugars, provide empty calories, and do not offer the same satiety as solid foods. Regular consumption of sugary beverages can lead to weight gain and an increased risk of obesity-related diseases.

5. **High-fat foods:** Diets high in unhealthy fats, such as saturated and trans fats, can contribute to weight gain and obesity. Foods like fried foods, fatty cuts of meat, full-fat dairy products, and processed snacks often contain high levels of unhealthy fats. These fats are calorie-dense and can lead to weight gain when consumed in excess.

6. **Ultra-processed foods:** Ultra-processed foods, which are highly manipulated and contain additives, are often high in calories, unhealthy fats, added sugars, and salt. These foods are designed to be convenient and hyper-palatable, making them easy to overconsume. Regular consumption of ultra-processed foods has been associated with obesity and poor health outcomes.

7. **Lack of dietary diversity:** Diets lacking in variety and primarily composed of energy-dense, nutrient-poor foods can contribute to weight gain and obesity. By not including a range of fruits, vegetables, whole grains, and lean proteins, individuals may miss out on essential nutrients while consuming excessive calories.

8. **Emotional and mindless eating:** Emotional eating, where individuals turn to food for comfort or as a coping mechanism, can contribute to weight gain. Mindless eating, often driven by distractions or eating quickly, can lead to overconsumption and a lack of awareness of fullness cues.

9. **Food marketing and availability:** The promotion and easy accessibility of unhealthy foods are significant contributors to obesity. Food marketing often targets children and can influence food preferences and choices. Additionally, the increased availability and aggressive promotion of fast food and unhealthy snacks contribute to their overconsumption.

10. **Socioeconomic factors:** Disparities in obesity rates exist across different socioeconomic groups. Lower-income communities often have limited access to affordable, nutritious foods, known as food deserts, while being surrounded by a higher density of fast food and convenience stores. This lack of access to healthy options can contribute to poor dietary choices and an increased risk of obesity.

In conclusion, several factors contribute to obesity, with diet playing a crucial role. Consuming energy-dense, nutrient-poor foods, larger portion sizes, high amounts of added sugars, unhealthy fats, and ultra-processed foods are key contributors. Alongside dietary factors, other aspects such as emotional eating, food marketing, and socioeconomic disparities further compound the issue. Addressing these factors through promoting healthier eating habits, improving food environments, and ensuring access to nutritious options can play a vital role in preventing and reducing obesity.

Obesity in foods can be caused by various factors. Here are some tips, causes, functions, advantages, and disadvantages that related to the issue:

Tips to Address Obesity in Foods:

1. **Focus on portion control:** Watch your serving sizes to avoid overeating.
2. **Choose whole, unprocessed foods:** Opt for fruits, vegetables, lean proteins, and whole grains.
3. **Read food labels:** Pay attention to the nutritional content and avoid products high in added sugars, unhealthy fats, and sodium.
4. **Cook at home:** Preparing your meals gives you control over ingredients and portion sizes.
5. **Reduce added sugar intake:** Limit consumption of sugary beverages, desserts, and processed foods.
6. **Be mindful of cooking methods:** Choose healthier options like grilling, steaming, or baking rather than deep-frying.
7. **Increase physical activity:** Regular exercise aids in weight management and overall health.

8. **Drink plenty of water:** Hydration helps promote satiety and reduce excessive snacking.

9. **Limit eating out:** Restaurant meals often contain hidden calories and larger portion sizes.

10. **Seek professional advice:** Consult a registered dietitian or nutritionist for personalized guidance and meal planning.

Causes of Obesity in Foods:

1. **High calorie content:** Foods that are high in calories contribute to weight gain.

2. **Excess fat and sugar:** Foods with high levels of unhealthy fats and added sugars can promote obesity.

3. **Processed and fast foods:** These types of foods are often nutrient-poor and calorie-dense.

4. **Portion sizes:** Large portion sizes lead to increased calorie intake.

5. **Lack of fruits and vegetables:** A diet lacking in these essential food groups can contribute to weight gain.

6. **Sedentary lifestyle:** Lack of physical activity combined with poor dietary choices can lead to obesity.

7. **Marketing and advertising:** The promotion of unhealthy foods can influence consumer choices.

8. **Economic factors:** Financial constraints may limit access to healthier food options.

9. **Genetics:** Certain genetic factors can predispose individuals to obesity.

10. **Emotional eating:** Using food as a means of coping with emotions can lead to overeating.

Functions of Obesity in Foods:

1. **Satiation:** Some foods that contribute to obesity may offer a feeling of fullness, temporarily satisfying hunger.
2. **Pleasure response:** High-calorie, sugary, and fatty foods can trigger the brain's reward system, leading to feelings of pleasure.
3. **Energy source:** Foods high in calories provide the body with energy.
4. **Taste enhancement:** Unhealthy ingredients like salt, sugar, and unhealthy fats can enhance the taste of foods.
5. **Convenience:** Fast foods and processed snacks are quick and accessible options, making them attractive to many.
6. **Preservation:** Certain unhealthy ingredients and additives extend the shelf life of processed foods.
7. **Cost-effectiveness:** Some calorie-dense, unhealthy foods are cheaper and more readily available compared to healthier alternatives.
8. **Socialization:** Eating foods that contribute to obesity is often associated with social gatherings and celebrations.
9. **Emotional comfort:** Indulging in certain foods may provide a temporary feeling of comfort during emotional distress.
10. **Habitual consumption:** Some individuals develop a habit of consuming foods high in calories, leading to obesity.

Advantages of Addressing Obesity in Foods:

1. **Improved health:** Addressing obesity in foods promotes better overall health and reduces the risk of various medical conditions.

2. **Weight management:** Balanced food choices help manage weight and prevent obesity.

3. **Increased energy levels:** Optimal nutrition supports energy levels required for daily activities.

4. **Better cardiovascular health:** A healthy diet reduces the risk of heart disease, high blood pressure, and other cardiovascular issues.

5. **Enhanced mental well-being:** Proper nutrition positively impacts cognitive function and mood.

6. **Reduced risk of diabetes:** Healthy eating habits contribute to the prevention and management of diabetes.

7. **Improved digestion:** A balanced diet rich in fiber content supports a healthy digestive system.

8. **Enhanced immune function:** Adequate nutrition strengthens the immune system, reducing the risk of infections and illnesses.

9. **Positive body image:** A healthy diet promotes self-confidence and a positive body image.

10. **Longevity:** Proper nutrition reduces the risk of premature death and increases life expectancy.

Disadvantages of Obesity in Foods:

1. **Increased risk of chronic diseases:** Obesity contributes to a higher risk of conditions like diabetes, cardiovascular diseases, and certain cancers.
2. **Reduced mobility:** Excessive weight gain can lead to limited physical mobility and joint issues.
3. **Decreased quality of life:** Obesity can negatively impact mental well-being, self-esteem, and overall quality of life.
4. **Financial burden:** Treating obesity-related health issues can lead to increased healthcare costs for individuals and society.
5. **Social stigma and discrimination:** Obese individuals may face unfair judgment and discrimination in various aspects of life.
6. **Reduced fertility:** Obesity can negatively affect fertility and reproductive health.
7. **Increased surgical risks:** Obesity poses challenges in performing surgeries and increases the risk of complications.
8. **Lowered immune function:** Obesity impairs immune function, leading to higher susceptibility to infections.
9. **Negative impact on sleep:** Obesity is associated with sleep disorders such as sleep apnea, which can affect overall well-being.
10. **Environmental impact:** The production and disposal of unhealthy food options can contribute to environmental degradation.

Addressing the causes and consequences of obesity in foods requires a multifaceted approach involving education, awareness, and policy interventions to promote healthier dietary practices.

CHAPTER 4: Source Of Overweight Prevention.

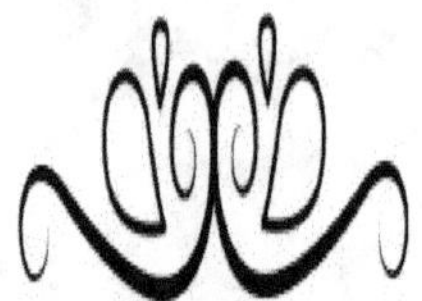

Source for Overweight Prevention.

Obesity prevention is a critical public health issue as the prevalence of obesity continues to rise worldwide. This summary will provide key sources and strategies for preventing obesity.

1. **Healthy Eating:** A balanced diet plays a fundamental role in obesity prevention. Encouraging the consumption of whole, unprocessed foods that are rich in nutrients, such as fruits, vegetables, whole grains, lean proteins, and healthy fats, is essential. Promoting healthy eating habits early in life through education and awareness campaigns is crucial for long-term prevention.

2. **Physical Activity:** Regular physical activity is essential for maintaining a healthy weight and preventing obesity. Encouraging individuals to engage in at least 150 minutes of moderate-intensity exercise per week can have significant health benefits. Promoting physical activity at schools,

workplaces, and communities can contribute to increased participation and a more active lifestyle.

3. **Early Childhood Intervention:** Recognizing the importance of early childhood in obesity prevention is essential. Effective strategies include promoting breastfeeding, introducing a variety of nutritious foods during infancy, limiting television/screen time, and ensuring high-quality early childhood education that includes nutrition and physical activity components.

4. **Community Interventions:** The environment plays a crucial role in shaping behaviors related to diet and physical activity. Creating communities that support healthy behaviors is essential for obesity prevention. This can include implementing policies to increase access to affordable healthy foods, creating safe and accessible recreational areas, and implementing bike-friendly and walkable infrastructure.

5. **School-Based Interventions:** Schools provide an ideal setting for obesity prevention interventions. Strategies can include offering nutritious meals and snacks, providing nutrition education, incorporating physical activity into the curriculum, and creating supportive environments that promote healthy behaviors.

6. **Policy and Advocacy:** Government policies and advocacy efforts can significantly impact obesity prevention. Implementing policies that regulate food marketing to children, mandating nutrition labeling, supporting menu labeling in restaurants, and implementing taxes on sugary

beverages are effective strategies to discourage unhealthy dietary choices.

7. **Media and Marketing Influence:** The media and marketing industries play a significant role in shaping individuals' food choices. By promoting healthier products and discouraging the marketing of unhealthy foods to children, we can create a healthier food environment.

8. **Health Education and Promotion:** Effective health education and promotion campaigns can raise awareness about the importance of healthy eating and physical activity. Utilizing various media platforms, social marketing techniques, and targeting diverse populations can help disseminate accurate information and motivate behavior change.

9. **Healthcare Providers' Role:** Healthcare providers have a critical role in obesity prevention. Through routine screenings, counseling on nutrition and physical activity, and referral to specialized services when necessary, healthcare professionals can play an important role in promoting healthy lifestyles.

10. **Research and Surveillance:** Ongoing research and surveillance are essential for understanding the complex factors contributing to obesity and evaluating the effectiveness of prevention strategies. Continuously monitoring obesity rates and associated risk factors can inform policy development and intervention efforts.

In conclusion, obesity prevention requires a comprehensive approach that addresses individual behaviors, community environments, policies, and societal norms. By implementing evidence-based strategies across multiple sectors, we can work towards reducing the prevalence of obesity and improving overall population health.

Sources.

Here are some sources you can refer to for information on obesity prevention:

1. **World Health Organization (WHO):** The WHO provides comprehensive guidelines and resources on obesity prevention, including tips, causes, functions, advantages, and disadvantages. You can visit their website at www.who.int.

2. **Centers for Disease Control and Prevention (CDC):** The CDC offers valuable information on obesity prevention, including tips for individuals, families, and communities. Their website at www.cdc.gov has numerous resources to help combat obesity.

3. **National Institute of Diabetes and Digestive and Kidney Diseases (NIDDK):** The NIDDK, a part of the National Institutes of Health, focuses on research and education related to obesity prevention and management. At www.niddk.nih.gov, you can find evidence-based information on causes, prevention strategies, and more.

4. **American Heart Association (AHA):** AHA emphasizes the link between obesity and cardiovascular health. Their website at www.heart.org provides reliable information on obesity

prevention tips, causes, functions, and overall advantages of maintaining a healthy weight.

5. **Mayo Clinic:** Mayo Clinic offers comprehensive resources on health and wellness, including obesity prevention. Visit www.mayoclinic.org for expert advice, tips, and causes related to obesity prevention.

6. **National Heart, Lung, and Blood Institute (NHLBI):** NHLBI focuses on research and education related to heart, lung, and blood disorders, including obesity. Their website at www.nhlbi.nih.gov provides evidence-based information on obesity prevention strategies and the advantages of maintaining a healthy weight.

7. **American Academy of Pediatrics (AAP):** AAP provides guidance on obesity prevention in children and adolescents. Visit www.aap.org for valuable resources and tips specifically tailored to child and adolescent health.

8. **Harvard University School of Public Health:** Harvard's School of Public Health offers evidence-based information and resources on obesity prevention. Their website at www.hsph.harvard.edu provides useful tips, functions, and advantages associated with maintaining a healthy weight.

9. **American Obesity Association (AOA):** AOA advocates for obesity prevention and offers resources on their website at www.obesity.org. They provide information on causes, prevention strategies, and potential disadvantages of obesity.

10. **WebMD:** WebMD is a popular health website that covers various topics, including obesity prevention. Their website at www.webmd.com offers a wide range of articles, tips, and

expert advice on causes, functions, advantages, and disadvantages associated with obesity prevention.

Remember to critically evaluate information from these sources and consult healthcare professionals for personalized advice. Obesity prevention encompasses various strategies and practices aimed at reducing the prevalence of obesity in individuals and communities. Here are the requested of some tips, causes, functions, advantages, and disadvantages related to obesity prevention.

Tips for Obesity Prevention:

1. Maintain a balanced diet with a focus on whole foods, fruits, vegetables, and lean proteins.
2. Engage in regular physical activity that combines aerobic exercise and strength training.
3. Limit the intake of sugary beverages, processed foods, and fast food.
4. Practice portion control and mindful eating to help manage calorie intake.
5. Get sufficient sleep to support healthy metabolism and hormone regulation.
6. Manage stress levels through techniques like meditation, yoga, or counseling.
7. Limit screen time and engage in outdoor activities to promote an active lifestyle.
8. Create a supportive environment at home and work that promotes healthy habits.

9. Seek support from healthcare professionals or weight management programs if needed.

10. Educate yourself and others about the risks and consequences of obesity.

Causes of Obesity:

1. Poor dietary choices and overconsumption of high-calorie, low-nutrient foods.

2. Sedentary lifestyle and lack of physical activity.

3. Genetics and family history of obesity.

4. Psychological factors like stress or emotional eating.

5. Environmental factors like easy access to unhealthy foods and built-in surroundings that discourage physical activity.

6. Certain medical conditions and medications that contribute to weight gain.

7. Hormonal imbalances, such as hypothyroidism or polycystic ovary syndrome.

8. Lack of education and awareness about healthy eating and lifestyle choices.

9. Socioeconomic factors, including limited access to nutritious food and resources for physical activity.

10. Cultural factors and societal norms that promote unhealthy eating behaviors.

Functions of Obesity Prevention:

1. Creating awareness about the risks associated with obesity-related conditions such as diabetes, cardiovascular diseases, and certain cancers.
2. Promoting healthy eating habits and encouraging the consumption of a nutrient-dense diet.
3. Encouraging regular physical activity to improve overall fitness and maintain a healthy weight.
4. Providing resources for individuals to make informed choices about their diet and lifestyle.
5. Implementing policies that regulate the marketing and availability of unhealthy foods.
6. Collaborating with schools, workplaces, and community organizations to establish healthy environments.
7. Conducting research to understand the root causes of obesity and develop effective prevention strategies.
8. Offering counseling and support to individuals struggling with weight management.
9. Empowering individuals through education and skills development.
10. Advocating for policies that address social inequalities and improve access to nutritious food and safe physical activity spaces.

Advantages of Obesity Prevention:

1. Improved overall health and wellbeing of individuals and communities.

2. Reduction in the risk of chronic diseases associated with obesity.
3. Increased productivity and reduced healthcare costs.
4. Improved self-esteem and body image.
5. Enhanced physical fitness and mobility.
6. Better mental health outcomes, including reduced risk of depression and anxiety.
7. Lower burden on healthcare systems and resources.
8. Improved quality of life for individuals and families.
9. Prevention of obesity-related disabilities and complications.
10. Promotion of healthier habits and behaviors across different age groups.

Disadvantages of Obesity Prevention:

1. The complex nature of obesity makes prevention challenging.
2. Implementation of prevention strategies requires significant effort and resources.
3. Societal and cultural resistance to change can hinder progress.
4. There may be conflicting information and confusion about the effectiveness of certain prevention approaches.
5. The impact of prevention efforts may take time to manifest, requiring long-term commitments.
6. Effectiveness of prevention strategies may vary based on individual factors.
7. There may be challenges in reaching marginalized or underserved populations.

8. Emotional and psychological barriers may hinder individuals from seeking or adhering to prevention strategies.

9. Prevention efforts may face opposition from industries profiting from unhealthy products.

10. Lack of policy support and public funding may limit the reach and impact of prevention initiatives.

It's important to note that the effectiveness of obesity prevention may vary for individuals, and a comprehensive approach involving multiple stakeholders is crucial for long-term success.

CHAPTER 5: Steps to Follow If You're Obese or Overweight.

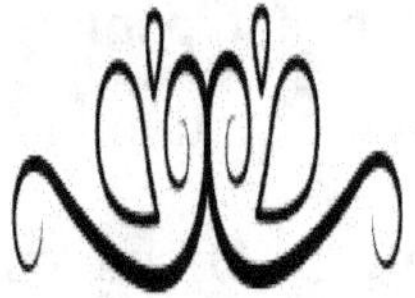

Steps to Follow If You're Obese or Overweight.

Being obese or overweight can have a significant impact on your overall health and quality of life. However, with the right approach and lifestyle changes, you can take control of your weight and improve your well-being. In this article, we will discuss the steps you can follow if you're obese or overweight, providing a comprehensive guide to help you achieve your weight loss goals.

Step 1: Understand Your Goals and Motivation.

Before embarking on any weight loss journey, it is crucial to identify and understand your goals. Are you looking to lose weight for aesthetic reasons, or do you have specific health concerns? Understanding your motivations will help keep you focused and committed throughout the process.

Step 2: Consult with Your Healthcare Professional.

It is wise to consult with your healthcare professional before starting any weight loss plan. They can help assess your overall health, provide guidance, and ensure that your weight loss strategy is safe and suitable for your specific needs.

Step 3: Set Realistic and Attainable Goals.

When setting weight loss goals, it is important to be realistic and consider your current health condition. Aim for gradual, sustained weight loss rather than quick fixes, as this is both healthier and more likely to lead to long-term success.

Step 4: Create a Balanced Diet Plan.

A well-balanced diet is fundamental to weight loss. Focus on consuming nutrient-dense foods such as fruits, vegetables, lean proteins, whole grains, and healthy fats. Avoid excessive sugar, saturated fats, and processed foods. Consider working with a registered dietitian who can develop a personalized meal plan to fit your needs and preferences.

Step 5: Practice Portion Control.

Portion control plays a vital role in weight management. Pay attention to your body's hunger signals and try to eat until you are comfortably full, rather than overeating. Using smaller plates and bowls can help control portion sizes and prevent overindulgence.

Step 6: Stay Hydrated.

Often, people mistake thirst for hunger and end up consuming unnecessary calories. Stay adequately hydrated by drinking plenty of water throughout the day. Water not only keeps you hydrated but can also help reduce cravings and promote a feeling of fullness.

Step 7: Include Regular Exercise.

Regular physical activity is essential for weight loss and overall health. Engage in a combination of aerobic exercises such as walking, running, swimming, or cycling, as well as strength training exercises to build muscle and boost metabolism. Aim for at least 150 minutes of moderate-intensity exercise or 75 minutes of vigorous exercise per week, as recommended by health experts.

Step 8: Find Support and Accountability.

Seeking support from family, friends, or joining a weight loss support group can significantly increase your chances of success. Surround yourself with individuals who have similar goals, as they can provide encouragement, motivation, and accountability.

Step 9: Manage Stress and Emotional Eating.

Many individuals turn to food for comfort when stressed or experiencing negative emotions. Finding healthy ways to manage stress, such as practicing mindfulness, engaging in hobbies, meditating, or seeking professional help, can help prevent emotional eating and support healthier coping mechanisms.

Step 10: Monitor Progress and Make Adjustments.

Regularly track your progress to stay motivated and identify areas for improvement. Use tools such as a food diary, weight tracker, or mobile applications to monitor your eating habits, physical activity, and weight loss journey. If faced with challenges or plateaus, be willing to adapt your approach and make necessary adjustments to your plan.

Remember, weight loss is a journey that requires patience and persistence. Embrace the process, stay consistent with healthy habits, and celebrate small victories along the way. With time, dedication, and the right support system, you can achieve a healthier weight and improve your overall well-being.

If you find yourself struggling with obesity or being overweight, there are several steps you can follow to make positive changes in your life and improve your overall health. Here is a summary of these steps, along with 10 tips, causes, factors, benefits, advantages, and disadvantages associated with addressing weight issues.

Steps to Follow If You're Obese or Overweight:

1. **Set realistic goals:** Begin by setting achievable goals for weight loss, such as aiming for a sustainable rate of 1-2 pounds per week.

2. **Consult a healthcare professional:** Seek guidance from a healthcare professional who can evaluate your overall health, provide personalized advice, and monitor your progress.

3. **Create a balanced and nutritious diet:** Focus on consuming a variety of whole, unprocessed foods, including fruits, vegetables, lean proteins, whole grains, and healthy fats, while limiting the intake of sugary and processed foods.

4. **Practice portion control:** Be mindful of your portion sizes to prevent overeating and ensure a calorie deficit that promotes weight loss.

5. **Stay hydrated:** Drink an adequate amount of water each day, as it can help control appetite, boost metabolism, and support overall health.

6. **Engage in regular physical activity:** Incorporate at least 150 minutes of moderate-intensity aerobic exercise or 75 minutes of vigorous exercise into your weekly routine, along with strength training exercises to build lean muscle mass.

7. **Get enough sleep:** Aim for 7-8 hours of quality sleep each night, as it plays a crucial role in weight management and overall well-being.

8. **Manage stress levels:** Find healthy coping mechanisms to handle stress, such as meditation, yoga, or engaging in hobbies, as stress can lead to emotional eating and weight gain.

9. **Seek social support:** Surround yourself with a supportive network of family and friends who can help you stay motivated and accountable on your weight-loss journey.

10. **Monitor and track your progress:** Keep a record of your food intake, exercise routine, and any changes in your weight to identify patterns and adjust your plan accordingly.

Tips for Addressing Obesity or Being Overweight:

1. Gradually incorporate healthy changes into your lifestyle rather than opting for crash diets or extreme exercise routines.

2. Stay consistent with your healthy habits even when progress seems slow. Sustainable weight loss takes time.

3. Find physical activities that you enjoy to increase your chances of sticking to an exercise routine.

4. Make use of technology, such as mobile apps or fitness trackers, to help monitor your calorie intake, track your exercise, and stay motivated.

5. Seek professional guidance from a registered dietitian or nutritionist to create a personalized meal plan that meets your nutritional needs.

6. Practice mindful eating by savoring each bite and paying attention to your body's hunger and fullness cues.

7. If emotional eating is a challenge, try finding alternative ways to cope with emotions, such as journaling or talking to a therapist.

8. Consider joining support groups or weight-loss programs to connect with others facing similar challenges and receive additional guidance and motivation.

9. Be kind to yourself and focus on the progress you make, rather than solely focusing on the number on the scale.

10. Remember that weight loss is not the sole determinant of good health. Focus on overall well-being and making sustainable lifestyle changes rather than obsessing over a specific weight goal.

Causes of Obesity or Being Overweight:

1. **Poor diet:** Consuming a diet high in processed foods, added sugars, and unhealthy fats can contribute to weight gain.

2. **Sedentary lifestyle:** Lack of physical activity and prolonged periods of sitting or inactivity can lead to weight gain.

3. **Genetics:** Some individuals may be genetically predisposed to obesity or have a slower metabolism, making it more challenging to maintain a healthy weight.

4. **Environment:** Living in an obesogenic environment where unhealthy food options are readily available and physical activity is limited can contribute to weight gain.

5. **Emotional factors:** Stress, depression, or other emotional factors can trigger emotional eating and lead to weight gain as a coping mechanism.

6. **Medical conditions:** Certain medical conditions, such as hypothyroidism or polycystic ovary syndrome (PCOS), can contribute to weight gain or make weight loss more difficult.

7. **Medications:** Some medications, such as certain antidepressants or corticosteroids, can cause weight gain as a side effect.

8. **Lack of sleep:** Inadequate sleep or poor sleep quality can disrupt hormones related to appetite regulation, leading to weight gain.

9. **Age:** Metabolism naturally slows down as we age, making it easier to gain weight and harder to lose it.

10. **Poor stress management:** High levels of chronic stress can increase cortisol levels and promote weight gain, particularly around the abdominal area.

Factors Influencing Obesity or Being Overweight:

1. **Caloric imbalance:** Consuming more calories than you burn on a regular basis leads to weight gain.

2. **Socioeconomic factors:** Limited access to healthy food options, lower education levels, and lower income can contribute to higher rates of obesity.

3. **Cultural and societal influences:** Cultural norms, such as larger portion sizes or frequent indulgence in high-calorie foods, can contribute to weight gain.

4. **Advertising and marketing:** Constant exposure to food advertisements promoting unhealthy options can impact eating behaviors and contribute to weight gain.

5. **Family dynamics:** Genetics, as well as shared eating and exercise habits within families, can play a role in obesity.

6. **Childhood experiences:** Adverse childhood experiences, including abuse or neglect, can increase the risk of obesity later in life.

7. **Eating behaviors:** Emotional eating, binge eating, or eating in response to external cues (e.g., advertisements or social gatherings) can contribute to weight gain.

8. **Food addiction:** Some individuals may develop an addiction to certain foods, leading to overconsumption and weight gain.

9. **Sleep patterns:** Disrupted sleep patterns or inadequate sleep can affect hormonal regulation, increasing the risk of weight gain.

10. **Mental health conditions:** Depression, anxiety, or other mental health conditions can impact eating behaviors and lead to weight gain or difficulties in weight management.

Benefits of Addressing Obesity or Being Overweight:

1. **Reduced risk of chronic diseases:** Weight loss can significantly decrease the risk of developing chronic conditions like heart disease, type 2 diabetes, and certain cancers.

2. **Improved cardiovascular health:** Losing excess weight can lower blood pressure and improve heart health.

3. **Enhanced mobility:** Weight loss can increase mobility and reduce joint pain, allowing for more physical activity and a better quality of life.

4. **Better sleep quality:** Shedding pounds can alleviate sleep apnea and improve the quality of sleep.

5. **Increased energy levels:** Losing weight can boost energy levels, making day-to-day activities feel less strenuous.

6. **Improved mental health:** Weight loss can positively impact self-esteem and body image, leading to improved mental well-being.

7. **Enhanced fertility:** Weight loss can improve fertility and increase the chances of a healthy pregnancy.

8. **Reduced medication reliance:** Addressing weight issues may decrease or eliminate the need for certain medications used to manage weight-related conditions.

9. **Improved digestion:** Weight loss can alleviate digestive issues like acid reflux and improve gut health.

10. **Enhanced overall quality of life:** Losing excess weight can lead to a higher overall quality of life, with increased confidence, improved mood, and a greater ability to engage in physical activities and social interactions.

Advantages of Addressing Obesity or Being Overweight:

1. **Increased life expectancy:** Maintaining a healthy weight can potentially extend your life expectancy.

2. **Improved self-image and body confidence:** Achieving a healthy weight can boost self-esteem and body confidence.

3. **Enhanced physical appearance:** Weight loss can lead to a more aesthetically pleasing physique.

4. **Better personal relationships:** Improved self-esteem and confidence can positively impact personal relationships.

5. **Increased productivity:** Improved physical and mental well-being resulting from weight loss can enhance productivity in various areas of life.

6. **Lower healthcare costs:** Addressing weight issues can lower healthcare costs associated with obesity-related conditions.

7. **Reduced risk of weight-related injuries:** Weight loss can decrease the risk of injuries caused by excess weight on joints or poor mobility.

8. **Enhanced athletic performance:** Achieving a healthy weight can improve athletic performance in various sports and physical activities.

9. **Ability to participate in more activities:** Losing weight can expand the range of activities and hobbies that can be enjoyed without physical limitations.

10. **Inspiring others:** By addressing your weight issues and achieving success, you can become an inspiration to others facing similar challenges, encouraging them to make positive changes in their own lives.

Disadvantages of Addressing Obesity or Being Overweight:

1. **Initial resistance to change:** The process of addressing weight issues may require significant lifestyle adjustments, which can be challenging and uncomfortable.

2. **Potential for plateaus:** Weight loss can sometimes plateau even with consistent efforts, which may be demotivating.

3. **Patience and determination required:** Sustainable weight loss takes time, and it requires commitment, consistency, and persistence.

4. **Social pressures and expectations:** Societal pressure or expectations regarding body image can add additional stress and negatively impact mental well-being.

5. **Emotional challenges:** The process of addressing weight can lead to emotional ups and downs, particularly if there are underlying issues related to body image or self-esteem.

6. **Need for ongoing maintenance:** Maintaining weight loss may require continued efforts and vigilance to prevent regain.

7. **Financial considerations:** Pursuing healthy eating habits or engaging in physical activities can incur additional costs, such as gym memberships or higher expenses for healthier food options.

8. **Potential for body image dissatisfaction:** Despite achieving weight loss goals, individuals may struggle with body image concerns or not feel satisfied with their appearance.

9. **Impact on social activities:** Adjusting lifestyle habits may affect socializing or participating in activities that revolve around food and sedentary behaviors.

10. **Potential for relapse:** For some individuals, weight regain can occur, which may require additional efforts to address and manage.

In summary, addressing obesity or being overweight involves a comprehensive approach that includes making lifestyle changes, seeking professional guidance, and staying committed to long-term goals. By following the tips and understanding the causes, factors, benefits, advantages, and disadvantages associated with weight management, individuals can embark on a transformative journey towards achieving a healthier weight and improving overall well-being.

CHAPTER 6: How To Create A Healthier & More Enjoyable Diet.

How To Create A Healthier & More Enjoyable Diet.

Creating a healthier and more enjoyable diet is a goal shared by many individuals seeking to improve their overall well-being. In this summary, I will provide you with key points to consider when embarking on this journey.

1. **Understand your nutritional needs:** It is crucial to comprehend your body's nutritional requirements, including macronutrients (carbohydrates, proteins, and fats) and micronutrients (vitamins and minerals). Consulting a healthcare professional or a registered dietitian can help you determine your specific needs.

2. **Incorporate a variety of whole foods:** Whole foods, such as fruits, vegetables, whole grains, lean proteins, and healthy fats, provide essential nutrients and minimize the intake of processed and refined foods. Strive for a colorful and diverse plate to ensure you obtain a wide range of nutrients.

3. **Portion control:** Pay attention to portion sizes to avoid overeating. Use smaller plates, bowls, and glasses, and be mindful of your hunger and satiety cues. Eating slowly and savoring each bite can also aid in portion control.

4. **Hydrate adequately:** Drinking sufficient water is vital for maintaining good health. It helps with digestion, nutrient absorption, and maintaining proper body temperature. Aim for at least 8 cups (2 liters) of water per day, and adjust this amount based on factors like activity level and climate.

5. **Limit added sugars and sweetened beverages:** Excessive intake of added sugars, like those found in sugary drinks, candies, and baked goods, can lead to weight gain, increased risk of chronic diseases, and energy crashes. Opt for natural sources of sweetness such as fruits, and choose water, herbal tea, or unsweetened beverages as alternatives.

6. **Reduce salt intake:** High sodium consumption can contribute to hypertension and other health issues. Be mindful of the salt content in processed foods, and try using herbs, spices, and other flavorings to enhance the taste of your meals.

7. **Plan and prepare meals:** Planning and prepping meals in advance can help you make healthier choices and avoid relying on convenience foods. Create a meal schedule, make a shopping list, and batch cook meals for the week. This can save time, money, and help you avoid unhealthy food options.

8. **Mindful eating:** Pay attention to your eating habits and make mealtime a mindful experience. Chew your food

thoroughly, eat at a table without distractions, and listen to your body's hunger and fullness signals.

9. **Exercise regularly:** Incorporating physical activity into your routine can complement a healthy diet. Engage in activities you enjoy, such as walking, swimming, or dancing, and aim for at least 150 minutes of moderate-intensity exercise per week.

10. **Seek support and guidance:** Changing eating habits can be challenging, so seek support from friends, family, or a support group. Consider working with a registered dietitian for personalized guidance and accountability.

Remember, creating a healthier and more enjoyable diet is a journey, and it is important to be patient with yourself. Gradual and sustainable changes tend to yield the best long-term results.

Tips.

Here are the tips to create a healthier and more enjoyable diets below.

1. **Eat a variety of fruits and vegetables:** Aim to include different types and colors of fruits and vegetables in your meals to ensure a wide range of nutrients.

2. **Incorporate whole grains:** Choose whole grains like brown rice, quinoa, and whole wheat bread to increase fiber intake and provide sustained energy.

3. **Include lean protein sources:** Opt for lean protein sources such as skinless poultry, fish, tofu, beans, and legumes to promote muscle growth and repair.

4. **Limit processed foods:** Minimize your intake of processed foods high in added sugars, unhealthy fats, and sodium, as they can negatively impact your health.

5. **Stay hydrated:** Drink plenty of water throughout the day to maintain proper hydration and support overall bodily functions.

6. **Cook at home:** Cooking your own meals allows you to control the ingredients and portion sizes, making your diet healthier and more enjoyable.

7. **Practice mindful eating:** Slow down while eating, savor each bite, and pay attention to your body's hunger and fullness cues.

8. **Reduce added sugars:** Be mindful of the added sugars in your diet and limit sugary beverages, sweets, and processed snacks.

9. **Include healthy fats:** Incorporate sources of healthy fats such as avocados, nuts, seeds, and olive oil for their cardiovascular and brain health benefits.

10. **Plan your meals:** Plan your meals in advance to ensure you have a balanced and nutritious diet, and consider meal prepping for added convenience.

Causes.

Now let's look at causes, benefits, and functions related to a healthier and more enjoyable diet:

1. Improved nutrient intake.

2. Reduced risk of chronic diseases.

3. Weight management.

4. Increased energy levels.

5. Enhanced mood and mental well-being.

6. Better digestion and gut health.

7. Improved immunity.

8. Healthy aging.

9. Reduced inflammation.

10. Enhanced athletic performance.

Benefits.

1. Increased vitality and overall well-being.

2. Weight loss or maintenance.

3. Improved cardiovascular health.

4. Lowered blood sugar levels.

5. Better sleep quality.

6. Stronger bones and teeth.

7. Clearer skin and healthier hair.

8. Better cognitive function and memory.

9. Reduced stress and anxiety.

10. Enhanced body composition

Functions.

1. Providing essential nutrients for growth and development.

2. Supporting cellular functions and tissue repair.

3. Regulating metabolism and energy production.

4. Aiding in digestion and nutrient absorption.

5. Supporting brain function and cognition.

6. Strengthening the immune system.

7. Promoting healthy hormone production.

8. Assisting in detoxification and elimination of waste.

9. Supporting healthy gut bacteria balance.

10. Providing antioxidants and reducing oxidative stress.

Remember, individual needs may vary, so it's essential to consult with a healthcare professional or registered dietitian for personalized advice based on your specific circumstances. How to create a healthier and more enjoyable diet.

Pros (Advantages/ Benefits):

1. Increased energy levels throughout the day.

2. Improved overall well-being and vitality.

3. Reduced risk of chronic diseases, such as heart disease and diabetes.

4. Better weight management and potential for weight loss.

5. Enhanced digestion and gut health.

6. Strengthened immune system for better resistance against illnesses.

7. Improved cognitive function and mental clarity.

8. Healthier skin, hair, and nails.

9. Better sleep quality and overall restfulness.

10. Improved mood and reduced stress levels.

Cons (Disadvantages/ Challenges):

1. Initial adjustment period as you adapt to new dietary changes.
2. Increased time and effort required for meal planning and preparation.
3. Possible higher costs associated with purchasing fresh and organic ingredients.
4. Social challenges during gatherings or dining out due to limited food options.
5. Cravings for unhealthy foods that may arise during the transition to a healthier diet.
6. Potential for nutrient deficiencies if the diet is not well-balanced or properly planned.
7. Difficulty in finding suitable options while traveling or eating on-the-go.
8. Possible resistance or lack of support from family, friends, or peers.
9. Potential for feeling overwhelmed with the abundance of dietary information available.
10. Personal taste preferences and potential dislike for certain healthier food choices.

It's important to note that these cons can be mitigated with proper planning, support, and gradually incorporating healthier choices into your lifestyle. Consulting with a healthcare professional or registered dietitian can provide tailored recommendations based on your specific needs and circumstances. Remember that the benefits of a healthier and more enjoyable diet generally outweigh the challenges, and it's worth investing in your long-term health and well-being.

How To Create A Healthier & More Enjoyable Diet.

Dieting can occasionally seem challenging, constrictive, and, to be perfectly blunt, burdensome. It doesn't have to be that way, though many of the typical Finding strategies to modestly modify your present living patterns rather than drastically altering them with the hope that doing so will result in weight loss may help you avoid the traps people make when dieting. By employing these methods, you ought to be on the road to a more fun and sustainable dieting strategy that works quickly.

The realistic and sustainable weight loss eating strategy.

Put an end to crash diets and begin a weight-loss plan that will enable you to lose weight gradually and safely. I should start by emphasizing that there is no one-size-fits-all method of nutrition for long-term weight loss. Despite some audacious marketing initiatives by some of the industry's major players in the health Industry, we must comprehend that losing weight requires dedication. Curating a lifestyle that is unique to you and your circumstances demands a conscious, consistent effort. I aim to offer some helpful advice on how to eat and exercise in the following paragraphs to successfully lose weight in the long term.

Recognizing BMR.

We should comprehend the fundamental concepts of Basal Metabolic Rate when it comes to weight loss (BMR). Simply put, our BMR measures the amount of energy that our body uses while at rest to perform tasks like digestion, blinking, and heart rate regulation. The ultimate goal of weight loss is to increase energy expenditure through regular resistance training and the growth of healthy muscle tissue Exercises with somewhat high intensity will aid in achieving that. You may use one of several online calculators to figure out your BMR, and once you know roughly how many calories your body needs each day at rest, you will be in a better position to plan your daily food intake. I'm not advocating that you track the calories in every meal for the rest of your life because the BMR equation is not an exact science. As you can control portion size and macronutrient ratios by having a general notion of how many calories are in each meal, it instead functions as a beginning point for a weight loss program. Eventually, you will increase your understanding of nutrition, specifically which food groups have the best nutritional value.

Low carbohydrate and high-fat macronutrient ratios.

It's simple to see how many of us can become confused about how much of each food category to eat given the abundance of web articles and recipe books recommended by health professionals. Low-fat diets are not as beneficial for weight loss as they have been portrayed to be in the mainstream media, although sample sizes are frequently small and study lengths rarely go beyond 12 months in the majority of the studies we have access to. Instead, doctors and nutritionists advise that meals high in dietary Fats and low carbohydrate diets are strongly linked to not just reduced inflammation and blood sugar control but also maintained weight loss. A low-carb, high-fat diet is a little more difficult to follow than it first appears. How much is considered low and high? By the meta-analyses previously mentioned, the studies under consideration classified low carbohydrate intake as comprising 33–47% of total daily intake. High fat consumption is not clearly defined, but studies repeatedly show that a Mediterranean diet rich in olive oil, fish, and nuts lowers fasting blood sugar levels, raises total cholesterol levels, and lowers blood pressure. Although there isn't much definitive evidence to back up ignoring standard dietary advice, it's obvious that the Government policies in the UK are ineffective. Experts in nutrition and cardiology like full-fat dairy products, oily fish, and meat in our meals rather than more carbohydrates. Here are some straightforward recommendations to promote lasting weight loss based on my experience dealing with individuals who want to lose weight. Schedule Meals Making the right decisions at mealtime can be aided by planning your meals out at least 24 hours in advance. Before doing out, you might desire a small snack, and subsequently, your body would benefit from consuming a high-quality protein source. Having these meals prepared lowers the likelihood of getting sidetracked and eating office cookies:

1. Avoid refined carbohydrates as much as possible.
2. An unprocessed, well-balanced diet that includes meat, fish, fruit, beans, nuts, seeds, and pulses will help our cells and hormones function normally.
3. Restricting refined carbs will support moderate energy levels and steady blood sugar levels.

4. They can be eliminated gradually over time to lessen the sense of depravity.

Consuming a colorful meal is a sure sign that it will be high in phytochemicals, vitamins, and minerals. Consume protein with each meal. The nutrition that supports strong muscle tissue is protein. Proteins of high quality can be found in meat, fish, lentils, beans, and dairy products. Be not afraid of fat A, D, E, and K vitamins certain vitamins are fat-soluble. This means that we must consume them through diet or supplements as our bodies are unable to create them on their own. Dietary fat enhances hormone regulation, bone density, and cell health. Avocados, olive oil, oily salmon, and almonds are good sources of the needed daily amount of fat. Regular exercise and weight lifting Your workout regimen should be focused on maintaining muscle mass and raising BMR. According to studies on the advantages of high-intensity interval training, if performed at the right intensity, you can achieve the same results as a long-duration steady-state exercise in half the time. Choose a high number of repetitions (12–15) with heavy weights when training the major muscular parts of your body in the gym (legs, chest, back, and shoulders   an   average   weight.

CHAPTER 7: What led to the rise of overweight ?

What led to the rise of overweight ?

The rise in obesity can be attributed to a combination of factors. Changes in dietary patterns, such as the increased consumption of processed and high-calorie foods, along with larger portion sizes, have contributed to weight gain. Sedentary lifestyles, where physical activity levels have decreased due to technology and urbanization, also play a role. Additionally, factors like genetic predisposition, socio-economic factors, and environmental influences can contribute to the rise in obesity. It's important to note that obesity is a complex issue with multiple causes, and addressing it requires a comprehensive approach involving education, policy changes, and individual lifestyle modifications.

Overweight treatment.

Overweight treatment is a complex and multifaceted topic that involves various approaches aiming to address the health implications of excess weight. In summarizing this broad subject, it is essential to cover key aspects such as lifestyle modifications, dietary interventions, physical activity, medical interventions, and psychological support.

The first pillar of overweight treatment is lifestyle modification, which includes changes in diet and physical activity patterns. Dietary interventions may involve reducing calorie intake, choosing nutrient-dense foods, and incorporating portion control. A balanced diet comprising carbohydrates, fats, and proteins, along with adequate intake of vitamins and minerals, is crucial. Specialized diets like the Mediterranean or DASH (Dietary Approaches to Stop Hypertension) diets have proven effective in promoting weight loss and improving overall health.

Physical activity plays a fundamental role in overweight treatment. Engaging in regular exercise not only aids in weight loss but also enhances cardiovascular function, strength, and mental well-being. Both aerobic exercises, such as walking, swimming, and cycling, and strength-training exercises, like weightlifting, are beneficial. Incorporating physical activity into daily routines can be achieved through activities such as taking the stairs instead of using elevators or dedicating time for structured exercise sessions.

In some cases, lifestyle modifications alone may not lead to significant weight loss or long-term maintenance. When appropriate, medical interventions can be considered. These may include prescription medications that help suppress appetite, decrease fat absorption, or increase metabolism. However, it is crucial to consult a healthcare professional to assess any potential risks, side effects, or contraindications associated with these medications.

In severe cases of obesity, when lifestyle modifications and medications have been unsuccessful, bariatric surgery may be considered. Bariatric surgery alters the digestive system, either through restriction (restrictive procedures) or a combination of restriction and malabsorption (malabsorptive procedures). Common types of bariatric surgery include gastric bypass, sleeve gastrectomy, and gastric banding. These procedures lead to significant weight loss and can improve or resolve obesity-related conditions such as type 2 diabetes, hypertension, and sleep apnea. However, surgery should always be approached as a last resort option after careful evaluation and consideration of potential risks and benefits.

Psychological support is another crucial component of overweight treatment. Emotional factors, such as stress, anxiety, and depression, can contribute to unhealthy eating behaviors and hinder weight loss efforts. Counseling, therapy, and support groups can help individuals address underlying psychological issues, develop coping strategies, and establish a positive relationship with food. Additionally, behavioral therapy can assist in identifying triggers for overeating, modifying unhealthy habits, and promoting sustainable lifestyle changes.

It is essential to approach overweight treatment holistically, considering the individual's overall health and well-being. Regular monitoring of weight, body composition, and relevant metabolic parameters such as blood pressure, blood sugar levels, and lipid profile is crucial to assess progress and guide treatment adjustments. Regular consultations with healthcare providers, dietitians, and exercise specialists can provide ongoing support and guidance throughout the treatment process.

In conclusion, overweight treatment involves a comprehensive approach that includes lifestyle modifications, dietary interventions, physical activity, medical interventions, and psychological support. This multifaceted approach aims to promote sustainable weight loss, improve overall health, and reduce the risk of obesity-related complications. Individualized treatment plans, tailored to the specific needs and preferences of each person, are key to long-term success in managing overweight and achieving optimal health.

Overweight treatment typically involves a combination of lifestyle changes, dietary modifications, increased physical activity, and, in some cases, medical interventions.

Tips.

Here are few tips for overweight treatment:

1. **Set realistic goals:** Establish achievable weight loss targets.
2. **Create a balanced diet:** Focus on nutritious, whole foods and portion control.

3. **Regular physical activity:** Engage in regular exercise to burn calories and improve overall fitness.

4. **Seek professional guidance:** Consult with healthcare professionals or registered dietitians.

5. **Monitor food intake:** Keep a food diary to track eating habits and identify areas for improvement.

6. **Stay hydrated:** Drink plenty of water to support metabolism and reduce calorie intake.

7. **Get support:** Join support groups or seek help from friends and family for motivation.

8. **Manage stress:** Find healthy ways to cope with stress and emotional eating.

9. **Sleep well:** Prioritize quality sleep as it can affect appetite and metabolism.

10. **Be patient and consistent:** Sustainable weight loss takes time and effort.

As for the factors leading to the rise in overweight treatment, they include the increasing prevalence of sedentary lifestyles, the availability of highly processed and calorie-dense foods, and changes in societal norms and behaviors regarding diet and physical activity. It's best to consult with healthcare professionals to evaluate specific benefits, functions, and potential drawbacks based on individual circumstances.

In summary, overweight treatment involves adopting a healthy lifestyle, seeking professional guidance, and making sustainable changes to achieve a healthy weight. It's important to approach weight loss with realistic expectations and focus on long-term well-being.

Factors contributing to the rise in obesity include:

1. **Changes in dietary patterns:** Increased consumption of processed and high-calorie foods.
2. **Larger portion sizes:** Serving sizes have grown over time, leading to increased calorie intake.
3. **Sedentary lifestyles:** Decreased physical activity due to technology and urbanization.
4. **Genetic predisposition:** Some individuals may be more prone to weight gain.
5. **Socio-economic factors:** Limited access to healthy foods and opportunities for physical activity.
6. **Environmental influences:** Built environments that discourage physical activity.
7. **Psychological factors:** Emotional eating and stress can contribute to weight gain.
8. **Marketing and advertising:** Promotion of unhealthy foods and beverages.
9. **Lack of nutritional education:** Limited knowledge about healthy eating habits.
10. **Medical conditions:** Certain medical conditions or medications can contribute to weight gain.

I provided some tips for managing weight below:

1. **Eat a balanced diet:** Focus on whole foods, fruits, vegetables, lean proteins, and whole grains.
2. **Portion control:** Be mindful of portion sizes to avoid overeating.
3. **Regular physical activity:** Engage in exercise or activities that you enjoy on a regular basis.
4. **Stay hydrated:** Drink water instead of sugary beverages to help control calorie intake.
5. **Practice mindful eating:** Pay attention to hunger and fullness cues while eating.
6. **Get enough sleep:** Aim for adequate sleep as it can affect appetite and metabolism.
7. **Manage stress:** Find healthy ways to manage stress rather than turning to food.
8. **Limit processed foods:** Minimize consumption of foods high in added sugars, fats, and sodium.
9. **Seek support:** Join support groups or find a weight loss program that suits your needs.
10. **Track progress:** Keep a record of your food intake and physical activity to monitor your progress.

The bottom line is that addressing obesity requires a comprehensive approach that involves making sustainable lifestyle changes, seeking professional guidance, and adopting a long-term perspective towards overall health and well-being. Overweight treatment has come about due to a multitude of factors, including societal concerns, health risks, and advancements in medical knowledge. Here are the requested 10 tips, causes, functions, advantages, and disadvantages related to overweight treatment:

Tips:

1. Focus on a balanced, nutrient-rich diet.
2. Engage in regular physical activity, such as exercises and workouts.
3. Set realistic weight loss goals and track progress.
4. Seek professional guidance from nutritionists or dietitians.
5. Limit consumption of sugary and processed foods.
6. Practice portion control and mindful eating.
7. Stay hydrated by drinking plenty of water.
8. Prioritize getting enough sleep and managing stress levels.
9. Incorporate lean proteins, fruits, vegetables, and whole grains into your meals.
10. Consider joining a support group or seeking psychological assistance to address emotional aspects related to weight management.

Causes:

1. Sedentary lifestyle, with reduced physical activity levels.
2. Unhealthy eating habits, including excessive consumption of calorie-dense foods.
3. Genetic factors and family history of overweight or obesity.
4. Psychological factors, such as emotional eating or using food as a coping mechanism.

5. Certain medical conditions and medications that can lead to weight gain.
6. Environmental factors, such as easy access to unhealthy food options.
7. Insufficient sleep or disrupted sleep patterns.
8. Hormonal imbalances, including conditions like polycystic ovarian syndrome (PCOS).
9. Age-related changes in metabolism, which can result in decreased calorie burning.
10. Socioeconomic factors, as overweight and obesity are more prevalent in disadvantaged populations.

Functions:

1. Developing personalized and tailored weight loss plans for individuals.
2. Providing nutritional counseling and education on healthy eating habits.
3. Recommending appropriate exercise regimens to boost metabolism and burn calories.
4. Monitoring progress through regular check-ups and body measurements.
5. Offering behavioral therapy to address emotional eating and develop coping mechanisms.
6. Providing access to weight management medications or supplements, when necessary.
7. Recommending bariatric surgeries for severely obese individuals.

8. Offering support groups and community programs for motivation and accountability.

9. Addressing underlying medical conditions that contribute to weight gain.

10. Promoting long-term lifestyle changes to sustain weight loss and prevent relapse.

Advantages:

1. Improved overall health and reduced risk of chronic diseases such as heart disease, diabetes, and certain cancers.

2. Enhanced self-esteem and body image.

3. Increased energy levels and improved physical fitness.

4. Better sleep quality and reduced symptoms of sleep disorders.

5. Improved mobility and decreased joint pain.

6. Lowered risk of complications during pregnancy and childbirth.

7. Improved fertility outcomes in individuals with obesity-related fertility issues.

8. Reduced healthcare costs associated with obesity-related conditions.

9. Improved mental well-being and reduced risk of depression and anxiety.

10. Longer life expectancy and improved quality of life.

Disadvantages:

1. Challenging and demanding journey, requiring dedication and effort.
2. Possibility of weight loss plateaus and fluctuations.
3. Potential nutrient deficiencies due to restrictive diets or inadequate supplementation.
4. Risk of regaining lost weight if long-term lifestyle changes are not maintained.
5. Potential side effects of weight loss medications or surgical interventions.
6. Emotional and psychological challenges during the weight loss process.
7. Social stigma and discrimination associated with overweight and obesity.
8. Limited accessibility to specialized weight loss programs in certain regions.
9. Financial burden of purchasing healthier food options or gym memberships.
10. Potential negative impact on body image and body acceptance, if not addressed holistically.

Please note that it's always advisable to consult with healthcare professionals for personalized advice and guidance regarding overweight treatment.

CHAPTER 8: Do Carbohydrates Affect How We Look?

Do Carbohydrates Affect How We Look?

Carbohydrates play a significant role in our diet and can significantly impact how we look. In this detailed explanation and summary, we will explore the effects of carbohydrates on our appearance, covering tips, causes, factors, benefits, advantages, and disadvantages.

1. Tips for Managing Carbohydrate Intake:

- Choose complex carbohydrates such as whole grains, vegetables, and legumes over simple carbohydrates like refined sugars.
- Balance your carbohydrate intake with other macronutrients like proteins and fats.
- Opt for low glycemic index carbs that release energy gradually, promoting stable blood sugar levels and preventing spikes in insulin.

- Monitor portion sizes to avoid consuming excessive carbohydrates.
- Diversify your carb sources to ensure a well-rounded nutrient intake.

2. Causes of Carbohydrate-Related Effects:

- Poor carbohydrate choices, such as consuming mostly refined sugars and processed foods, can lead to weight gain, inflammation, and skin issues.
- Overconsumption of carbohydrates compared to energy expenditure can result in weight gain and an undesirable appearance.
- Insufficient fiber intake from carbohydrates can lead to digestive problems and affect how we look.

3. Factors Influencing Carbohydrate Effects:

- **Metabolic rate:** Different individuals metabolize carbohydrates differently, impacting weight management and physical appearance.
- **Activity level:** Active individuals require more carbohydrates for energy, while sedentary people may need to control their carb intake to avoid weight gain.
- **Genetic factors:** Some individuals may have genetic predispositions that affect how their body responds to carbohydrate consumption.

- **Hormonal balance:** Hormonal imbalances can influence how our bodies store and utilize carbohydrates, affecting weight and appearance.

4. Benefits of Appropriate Carbohydrate Intake:

- **Energy source:** Carbohydrates provide the primary fuel for our bodies, supporting physical performance and cognitive function.
- **Muscle growth:** Adequate carbohydrate intake supports muscle glycogen replenishment, essential for muscle growth and recovery.
- **Satiety:** Carbohydrates contribute to the feeling of fullness, reducing the chances of overeating and supporting weight management.

5. Advantages of Carbohydrates for Appearance:

- **Healthy skin:** Complex carbohydrates, rich in fiber and nutrients, can improve skin health by reducing inflammation and promoting collagen synthesis.
- **Hair health:** Proper carbohydrate intake supports hair growth and strength through its influence on cell turnover and protein synthesis.
- **Nail health:** Carbohydrate-rich diets can aid in maintaining healthy nails by providing necessary nutrients for growth and integrity.

6. Disadvantages of Excessive Carbohydrate Consumption:

- **Weight gain:** Consuming more carbohydrates than needed can lead to weight gain due to the excess calories they provide.
- **Insulin resistance:** A diet high in refined carbohydrates can contribute to insulin resistance, potentially leading to metabolic disorders and an unhealthy appearance.
- **Inflammation:** Simple carbohydrates and processed foods can cause inflammation in the body, leading to skin issues like acne and redness.

In summary, managing carbohydrate intake is crucial for how we look. By following tips such as choosing complex carbohydrates, balancing macronutrients, and monitoring portion sizes, we can optimize their effects. Poor carbohydrate choices, overconsumption, and insufficient fiber intake can lead to weight gain, inflammation, and skin problems. Factors like metabolic rate, activity level, genetics, and hormonal balance also influence how carbohydrates affect appearance. However, appropriate carbohydrate intake offers numerous benefits, including energy, muscle growth, and satiety. Additionally, carbohydrates contribute to healthy skin, hair, and nails. Conversely, excessive carbohydrate consumption can lead to weight gain, insulin resistance, and inflammation. Thus, a balanced approach is essential in managing carbohydrate intake to positively impact how we look.

CHAPTER 9: The mystery of calories.

The mystery of calories.

The mystery of calories has long intrigued individuals seeking to understand the relationship between food, energy, and weight management. Calories are units of energy derived from the food we consume, and they play a crucial role in maintaining bodily functions and supporting physical activity. However, the concept of calories can be complex, and misconceptions abound.

To unravel the mystery, it is essential to comprehend the basics. Calories serve as the fuel that powers our bodies, providing energy for essential physiological processes, such as breathing, digestion, and circulation. The energy we expend during physical activity is also measured in calories. In simplistic terms, weight gain occurs when we consume more calories than we burn, while weight loss occurs when we burn more calories than we consume. This principle forms the foundation of calorie balance.

Understanding the calorie content of various foods is crucial for making informed dietary choices. Different foods contain different amounts of calories due to their macronutrient composition. Fats provide the most concentrated source of calories, followed by carbohydrates and proteins, each contributing a specific number of calories per gram. By being aware of the calorie content of foods, individuals can better manage their energy intake and optimize their weight goals.

However, calories are not the sole determinant of a healthy diet. Nutrient density, which refers to the number of essential nutrients a food contains relative to its calorie content, is equally important. Consuming nutrient-dense foods, such as fruits, vegetables, whole grains, and lean proteins, ensures that our bodies receive the necessary vitamins, minerals, and other beneficial compounds while keeping calorie intake in check. Relying solely on calorie counting without considering nutrient density may lead to an imbalanced diet lacking essential nutrients.

While understanding calories can be empowering, it is essential to strike a balance and avoid becoming overly fixated on numbers. Calorie awareness should not become an obsession or lead to unhealthy behaviors. Extreme or restrictive diets centered solely around calorie counting can lead to disordered eating patterns and a negative relationship with food. It is crucial to prioritize overall health and well-being rather than becoming solely focused on calories.

One common pitfall is the inaccurate estimation of calorie values. Food labels and databases provide approximate values, but factors such as cooking methods, food preparation, and individual variations can affect the actual caloric content. Additionally, the body's metabolism and energy expenditure are not solely determined by calorie intake but are influenced by various factors, including genetics, age, body composition, and activity level. Therefore, calorie counting should be viewed as an estimation rather than an exact science.

Calorie awareness can be a useful tool for weight management, allowing individuals to monitor and adjust their energy intake according to their goals. It promotes portion control and mindful eating, encouraging individuals to be more conscious of their food choices and eating habits. However, it is important to remember that weight management is a complex interplay of various factors, including genetics, lifestyle, and overall health. Consulting a registered dietitian or healthcare professional can provide personalized guidance and support.

The benefits of calorie awareness extend beyond weight management. By understanding calorie content, individuals can make informed choices about their dietary patterns and optimize their nutrition. It promotes a balanced approach to eating, emphasizing whole, unprocessed foods that provide essential nutrients while controlling calorie intake. Calorie awareness also increases self-awareness, allowing individuals to reflect on their eating behaviors and make positive changes.

However, there are potential drawbacks to calorie awareness that should be considered. Some individuals may develop an unhealthy obsession with numbers, fixating on calorie counting to the point of anxiety or distress. This can lead to an unhealthy relationship with food and detrimental effects on mental and emotional well-being. The complexity of accurately measuring calorie intake and the variability in calorie content due to cooking methods and food preparation can also pose challenges. It is essential to approach calorie awareness with a balanced mindset and prioritize overall health rather than solely focusing on numbers.

In conclusion, the mystery of calories lies in their intricate relationship with food, energy, and weight management. Understanding calories can be empowering, enabling individuals to make informed dietary choices, manage their weight, and optimize their nutrition. However, it is crucial to approach calorie awareness with balance and mindfulness, avoiding extremes and potential pitfalls. Prioritizing nutrient density and overall well-being, consulting professionals when needed, and adopting a holistic approach to health are key to unraveling the mystery and finding a sustainable, healthy lifestyle.

Here are some insights into the mystery of calories.

Tips:

1. **Understand calorie balance:** Weight loss occurs when calories consumed are fewer than calories burned.
2. **Focus on nutrient density:** Choose foods that are rich in nutrients relative to their calorie content.
3. **Read food labels:** Pay attention to serving sizes and calorie information to make informed choices.
4. **Cook at home:** Preparing meals allows better control over ingredients and portion sizes.
5. **Be mindful of portion sizes:** Use smaller plates and practice portion control to prevent overeating.
6. **Increase physical activity:** Regular exercise helps burn calories and improve overall health.
7. **Include fiber-rich foods:** Fiber promotes satiety and can help control calorie intake.
8. **Limit sugary beverages:** High in calories and low in nutritional value, these can contribute to weight gain.
9. **Be mindful of liquid calories:** Alcoholic beverages and high-calorie drinks can add up quickly.
10. **Seek professional guidance:** Consult with a registered dietitian for personalized advice and calorie management.

Benefits of understanding calories:

1. **Weight management:** Calorie awareness facilitates better control over weight gain or loss.
2. **Increased energy levels:** Balancing calorie intake with energy expenditure can help maintain energy levels.
3. **Improved nutrition:** Conscious calorie choices encourage the consumption of nutrient-rich foods.
4. **Enhanced portion control:** Understanding calorie content aids in appropriate portion sizes.
5. **Better food choices:** Calorie awareness promotes healthier selections and reduces reliance on processed foods.
6. **Increased self-awareness:** Knowing calorie content raises awareness of eating habits and patterns.
7. **Personalized approach:** Understanding individual calorie needs allows for tailored dietary plans.
8. **Fitness optimization:** Monitoring calorie intake supports fitness goals and performance.
9. **Long-term health benefits:** Maintaining a healthy weight through calorie management can reduce the risk of chronic diseases.
10. **Sustainable lifestyle changes:** Calorie awareness fosters long-term habits for a healthier lifestyle.

Functions of calories:

1. **Energy provision:** Calories provide the energy needed for bodily functions and physical activity.

2. **Metabolism support:** Calories fuel the metabolic processes that keep the body functioning.

3. **Growth and development:** Sufficient calories are crucial for growth, particularly in children and adolescents.

4. **Organ function:** Calories support the proper functioning of organs and systems in the body.

5. **Muscle maintenance:** Sustaining muscle mass requires adequate calorie intake.

6. **Body temperature regulation:** Calories provide energy for maintaining body temperature.

7. **Hormonal balance:** Sufficient calories help maintain a healthy hormonal balance.

8. **Brain function:** The brain relies on calories for optimal cognitive performance.

9. **Cell repair and maintenance:** Calories support cell renewal and repair processes in the body.

10. **Overall well-being:** Calories contribute to overall health and vitality.

Pros of calorie awareness:

1. Increased control over weight management.

2. Improved understanding of nutritional needs.

3. Empowerment to make informed food choices.

4. Flexibility in dietary planning.

5. Awareness of energy balance and expenditure.

6. Ability to personalize dietary approaches.

7. Greater awareness of portion sizes.

8. Opportunity for self-reflection and behavior change.

9. Potential for improved body composition.

10. Enhanced overall health and well-being.

Cons of calorie awareness:

1. Potential to foster an unhealthy obsession with numbers.
2. Overemphasis on quantity rather than quality of food.
3. Risk of developing disordered eating patterns.
4. Difficulty accurately measuring calorie intake.
5. Variability in calorie content due to cooking methods and food preparation.
6. Limited focus on other aspects of nutrition, such as nutrient density.
7. Potential for stress and anxiety related to tracking and monitoring calories.
8. Misinterpretation of calorie values leading to inaccurate estimations.
9. Perceived complexity of calorie counting.
10. Difficulty in maintaining long-term adherence.

Bottom line: Understanding calories can be a helpful tool in managing weight, making informed food choices, and promoting overall health. However, it's important to approach calorie awareness with balance, avoiding extremes and potential pitfalls. Individual needs and preferences should be considered, and professional guidance may be beneficial for personalized advice and support.

Tips:

1. **Track your calorie intake:** Keeping a food diary or using a calorie-tracking app can help you become aware of your calorie consumption.
2. **Eat whole, unprocessed foods:** These typically have fewer calories but are more nutrient-dense, promoting better overall health.
3. **Practice portion control:** Be mindful of serving sizes and try not to overeat.
4. **Eat mindfully:** Pay attention to your hunger and fullness cues, and avoid distractions while eating.
5. **Include protein in your meals:** Protein can increase satiety, helping you feel fuller for longer.
6. **Be aware of hidden calories:** Watch out for calorie-dense sauces, dressings, and sugary drinks, as they can contribute significantly to your daily intake.
7. **Stay hydrated:** Drinking water before meals can help curb appetite and prevent overeating.

8. **Incorporate regular physical activity:** Exercise can boost your metabolism and help burn calories.

9. **Get enough sleep:** Poor sleep can disrupt appetite hormones, leading to increased calorie intake.

10. **Seek support if needed:** If you struggle with managing your calorie intake or maintaining a healthy weight, consider reaching out to a registered dietitian or healthcare professional for guidance.

Causes:

1. **Overeating:** Consuming more calories than your body needs on a regular basis can lead to weight gain.

2. **Sedentary lifestyle:** Lack of physical activity can contribute to an imbalance between calories consumed and calories burned.

3. **Emotional eating:** Using food as a coping mechanism for stress, sadness, or other emotions can lead to excessive calorie intake.

4. **High-calorie processed foods:** Consuming a diet high in processed snacks, fast food, and sugary beverages can contribute to a calorie surplus.

5. **Lack of awareness:** Not paying attention to portion sizes or nutritional content can lead to unintentional overconsumption of calories.

6. **Genetic factors:** Some individuals may have a genetic predisposition to store calories more efficiently, making weight management challenging.

7. **Medications:** Certain medications may alter appetite, metabolism, or other factors related to calorie balance.

8. **Medical conditions:** Hormonal imbalances, such as an underactive thyroid, can affect metabolism and calorie utilization.

9. **Aging:** Metabolism naturally slows down with age, meaning fewer calories are needed to maintain weight.

10. **Social and environmental factors:** Food availability, cultural practices, and social settings can influence calorie consumption.

Functions:

1. **Energy production:** Calories provide the energy required for bodily functions, including physical activity, metabolism, and cellular processes.

2. **Maintenance of body temperature:** Calories contribute to heat production, helping to regulate body temperature.

3. **Organ function:** Calories are necessary for the proper functioning of organs like the heart, brain, liver, and kidneys.

4. **Muscle contraction:** Calories are utilized by muscles during movement and exercise.

5. **Growth and development:** Adequate calorie intake supports normal growth and development, especially in children and adolescents.

6. **Hormone production:** Certain hormones involved in metabolism and overall health are synthesized using energy from calories.

7. **Brain function:** The brain relies on calories to support cognitive function, memory, and overall mental well-being.

8. **Cell maintenance and repair:** Calories are needed for the maintenance and repair processes within cells.

9. **Immune system support:** Calories play a role in supporting a healthy immune system, helping to protect against illness and infection.

10. **Healthy skin, hair, and nails:** Adequate calorie intake supports the growth and maintenance of healthy skin, hair, and nails.

Advantages:

1. Provides energy for daily activities and exercise.
2. Helps in maintaining a healthy metabolism.
3. Supports organ function and overall health.
4. Can fuel athletic performance and muscle growth.
5. A well-balanced calorie intake can contribute to weight management goals.
6. Adequate calorie consumption can support proper growth and development in children and adolescents.
7. Can provide satiety and help prevent excessive hunger.
8. Promotes proper brain function and cognitive performance.
9. Supports the immune system and overall disease resistance.
10. Can positively impact physical appearance by maintaining healthy skin, hair, and nails.

Disadvantages:

1. Excessive calorie intake can contribute to weight gain and obesity.
2. High-calorie foods are often low in nutritional value, leading to nutrient deficiencies.
3. Regular consumption of calorie-dense foods can increase the risk of chronic diseases like heart disease and diabetes.
4. Restrictive calorie diets can lead to nutrient imbalances and inadequate intake of essential vitamins and minerals.
5. Focusing solely on calorie counting may neglect the quality of food consumed.
6. Obsession with calorie counting can lead to an unhealthy relationship with food and promote disordered eating behaviors.
7. Some calorie-dense foods, particularly highly processed ones, tend to be addictive and can result in overconsumption.
8. Drastic calorie restriction can slow down metabolism and make weight loss more challenging in the long term.
9. Strict calorie counting may be time-consuming and burdensome, potentially affecting social and mental well-being.
10. Calorie-focused diets often fail to account for individual differences in metabolic rate, body composition, and overall health.

Remember that individual needs and circumstances can vary, so it's essential to consult with a healthcare professional or registered dietitian for personalized advice on managing calories and maintaining a healthy lifestyle.

Taking Back Control.

Being proactive is usually a good idea. How many of us show up at lunchtime ravenous and unprepared? Usually, that's where issues arise. This is the rationale behind the daily uniforms. According to psychologists, we all have a limited capacity for decision-making, so by eliminating a straightforward option like what to dress, Mark is lowering the possibility of experiencing "decision fatigue" later in the day when working on more difficult tasks. From a nutritional standpoint, this can entail batch cooking on the weekends or hiring a food delivery service so that you can readily decline Susan's afternoon offer of cookies.

There just isn't any amount of accountability involved, which is why the majority of new year's resolutions fail. It is best to have a companion on board with you at all times one of the most important components of maintaining motivation and honoring your promise. A personal trainer could provide this accountability, or you could just tell your friends, family, and followers on social media about your strategy. Naturally, you should be doing this for your benefit, but getting support from friends, family, and/or a personal trainer who cares about your outcomes will be quite motivating. Anyone who wants to be successful at long-term weight management must first understand the distinction between hunger and appetite. While appetite typically refers to a hedonistic desire for food, hunger can be regarded as a physiological requirement to consume to maintain life. eating for energy efficiency and assistance Our basic perspective on nutrition ought to be optimum health. To navigate the various phases of dieting, determine the proper serving sizes, offer ongoing feedback, and help you raise your nutrition I.Q. along the way, expert guidance is invaluable. The essential components of any effective plan to encourage healthy weight loss and aid in long-term weight management are outlined in the list below:

- Engaging in at least 2-3 weekly workouts.
- Aim for 8000–10,000 steps per day.
- Sleeping for 7-9 hours per night.
- Consuming enough water for your body's needs.
- Eating a balanced diet that contains enough macro- and micronutrients.
- Supplementation, if required, to meet rising demands

Bringing everything together.

Losing weight might be a difficult notion for some people and can present many difficult roadblocks. Many of us are now suffering from the health decline brought on by long, sedentary workdays, hectic social schedules, and overindulging over holidays. Our "calories in" side of the equation are constantly shifting based on the demands we place on our bodies, and as the years pass, our inaction usually catches up with us. Before beginning a weight loss journey, one of your most essential assets will be understanding your "why." You may have just gotten engaged and are preparing for the big event. Or perhaps you're getting close to a big birthday and want to be in the best form of your life. Alternatively, you may be acting out of concern for your health because cardiovascular disease runs in your family. Whatever it may be, having this knowledge can help you get started, catch you if you fall, and keep you going all the way to the finish line. Whether you want to go solo or not, taking that first step is crucial.

Exposing the top three lies about calories and weight loss.

Every day it seems like a new headline is published claiming to have the "magic" solution to maintaining weight. What about the rest of us? For celebrities, the solution appears to be a personal trainer, chef, nutritionist, spiritual healer, and possibly a plastic surgeon. The reality is that effective weight management strategies: focus more on "math" and less on "magic." Fortunately, there isn't any algebra required, but you (or your smartphone) might need to perform some basic addition and subtraction to achieve a balance between the calories you take in and the calories you expend. It's crucial to comprehend calorie balance if you want to lose or maintain your weight. But despite the overwhelming body of research showing that calories are the key, there is still considerable misunderstanding and incorrect information around this issue. Here are the top 3 **myths** that the "Calorie Conundrum" is based on, according to the dietician I am.

MYTH #1: Calories from specific dietary sources help people lose weight more than calories from other sources.

FACT: Every calorie has the same effect on weight loss. Considering calories from proteins, carbs, and fat different? No matter what food source it comes from, a calorie is always a calorie. You still consume 100 calories whether you eat 100 calories of yogurt or 100 calories of candy. Although the body typically burns calories from carbohydrates first, followed by calories from protein, and then calories from fat, many widely adopted diets have placed more emphasis on limiting the quantity of fat, carbohydrate, or protein consumed than on urging people to pay attention to their overall calorie intake. In actuality, concentrating on eating a well-balanced macronutrient diet is what is most crucial. The USDA suggests that individuals, ages 19 and older, consume between 45 and 65 percent of their calories from carbohydrates, 10 and 35 percent from protein, and 20 and 35 percent from fat With this framework, it will be much simpler to follow this kind of diet for a longer period as opposed to switching to the next fad diet that restricts particular macronutrients. Numerous studies have looked at the effects of several diets, each with a different ratio of fat, protein, and carbohydrates, on weight loss and support the idea of eating a well-balanced macronutrient diet. Numerous studies have demonstrated that low-calorie diets and regular exercise lead to long-term weight loss regardless of the macronutrients that individuals in the study were instructed to take in the majority. The basic fact is that, regardless of the type of diet, weight reduction is similar for everyone who reduces their overall calorie consumption. It follows that All calories matter when it comes to weight management. Now, if you consider calories in terms of their nutritional value, not all calories are created equal. For instance, 100 calories from a candy bar won't offer as much protein and other essential nutrients as 100 calories from yogurt. Therefore, it's crucial to consider your entire, balanced diet when attempting to attain calorie balance for weight management and to make sure you're still getting the nutrients you need. For this reason, the ONLY strategy for long-term weight management is to consume a balanced diet that includes a range of foods and also satisfies your daily caloric demands.

MYTH #2: It is impossible to eat everything I want and stay within a healthy weight range.

FACT: Being conscious The BEST way to consume the food you want without expanding your girth is to control your portion sizes. Everybody has some foods that make losing or maintaining weight feel like our personal kryptonite. We decide to completely remove them from our pantries and confine them to our culinary fantasies because we feel helpless in the face of their enchantment. However, for long-term weight management and satisfaction, that is probably not the best course of action. I can eat the meals I prefer as long as I control the portion sizes, rather than fully abstaining from the things I enjoy. The word" (moderation) may sound cliche, but it is accurate. Having all of your favorite meals in moderation has far greater benefits Rather than committing to a "cleanse" of certain foods just to gorge on them later when depressive feelings take control, this strategy makes more sense. The bottom line is that you CAN have your cake and eat it too if you are attempting to maintain your weight, provided that your daily caloric intake and physical activity are in balance.

MYTH #3: Exercise doesn't aid in the control of weight.

FACT: Staying in balance can be achieved in large part through physical activity. Physical activity can have a significant impact on weight control if you are constantly consuming more calories than you need while trying to maintain your weight. Imagine your body as a fuel tank. Whenever you routinely fill you're If you consume more calories through food and drink than you expend through exercise, your body will be out of balance and you will put on weight. You should consume as many calories as your body expels each day if you're seeking to maintain your weight. The energy used to digest food, the energy used during physical activity, and the resting metabolic rate can all be divided into separate categories according to a scientific review. The term "metabolism" refers to the first two elements combined. The final element can be divided between daily activities like walking and organized exercise programs. We typically burn the most calories through metabolism, but we also burn more calories when we move more.

If you'd like If you want to lose weight, you should continuously consume fewer calories than your body requires each day and move more to burn off stored calories. While every person has different calorie requirements, in general, you need to reduce your calorie intake by about 500 calories per day or increase your physical activity for every pound of weight you wish to lose per week. This can be accomplished by switching to lower-calorie or calorie-free options or by consuming smaller portions of higher-calorie foods and beverages. Additionally, you can engage in a variety of physical activities that increase daily calorie expenditure and provide you with more food flexibility. Do you NEED to be physically active to maintain or lose weight? In theory, no, but Keep in mind that persons who exercise AND manage their diets have the most success at controlling their weight. There are restrictions on how much physical activity one can perform, particularly while trying to reduce weight, so exercise is only one part of the weight reduction equation. There is a limit to how much exercise a person can do safely and without being hurt, as there is with most activities. Finding an activity style (aerobic vs. aerobic) that suits your demands is crucial if you want to maintain a healthy, balanced weight.

Exercise and Diet Is A Calorie Myth.

We've all heard the conventional wisdom to eat healthier and exercise more to keep or reach a healthy weight. But what exactly does this mean? Exercise and diet are very ambiguous concepts for someone attempting to manage their health. This uncertainty creates a lot of traps that make it difficult or even impossible to accomplish one's goals. The power of a balanced diet is sometimes undervalued while the impact of exercise is frequently overestimated. Those who are trying to reduce weight find this to be particularly challenging. Continue reading for information you can utilize to advance your efforts and strengthen your health. Everything comes down to calories in the end. Your consumption and spending patterns have the strongest influence on body weight. In their attempts to lose weight or regulate their weight, many people get disheartened at this point. Let's be honest. People often don't want to worry about calories since they are dull. It is far simpler to put less emphasis on limitations and more emphasis on acting (i.e., working out). How else would you account for the spike in purchases of workout equipment around the New Year? There are countless reasons why exercise is important, but unless you frequently run marathons, its immediate impact on weight is negligible. Imagine you and your buddies are watching a movie late at night when they all decide to order pizza. While others devour three or four pieces, you're attempting to be more restrained good, so you decide to stop at two and have a glass of water. You even decide to "burn it off" the following morning by running three miles at the gym. The sad fact is that you only burned 300 calories—less than half of your indulgence—during all that running, which added up to roughly 600 calories (plus or less, depending on the pizza). If you keep doing that, it won't surprise you that despite your best efforts in the gym, so many people unintentionally put on the freshman. Considering that one mile of running burns roughly 100 calories (remember, this is just a rough estimate), it would take 35 miles of running to shed one pound of body fat. It's one mile a day for around a month, or if you're ambitious, 5 kilometers every day for a week. No one has time for that! However, reducing 500 calories a day for a week could be an alternative to losing this pound. All that is necessary for college students to do this is to give up a few poor habits. Choose oatmeal for 150 calories instead of the 450 in a muffin, and save another 200 calories by choosing water over an orange juice drink. You can do this even with nutritious foods. An orange, for instance, has about half as many calories as an apple. It would be tedious to keep track of every single calorie, therefore you don't need to.

merely being aware of too many calories and scanning It's simple to develop the habit of reading nutrition labels. Make a note of the items you eat most frequently and look up their nutritional facts; you only need to do this once, and the knowledge will stick with you to guide your decision-making. It's a numbers game when it comes to your weight, and what you can accomplish on an elliptical machine pales in comparison to the figures linked with eating. However, that does not imply that exercise is not crucial. One of the most crucial things you can do for your health is this. However, if I wanted to save 100 calories from my diet, I would much rather order my sandwich without mayo than run a mile more on the Stairmaster.

CHAPTER 10: The Roots Of overweight.

The Roots Of overweight.

Obesity is a global health issue that has reached epidemic proportions in recent decades. It is characterized by excessive body fat accumulation, resulting in various health complications such as cardiovascular diseases, diabetes, and certain types of cancer. Understanding the roots of obesity is crucial in order to effectively tackle this problem. In this essay, we will explore the various factors contributing to obesity and provide a comprehensive summary of its underlying causes.

One of the primary factors contributing to obesity is an unhealthy diet. The availability and consumption of highly processed, calorie-dense foods have dramatically increased in modern society. These foods are often high in sugars, unhealthy fats, and artificial additives, while lacking essential nutrients. The rise of fast-food chains, convenience foods, and food marketing targeted at children have further exacerbated the problem. Additionally, the increasing consumption of sugary beverages has played a significant role in the obesity epidemic.

Physical inactivity is another major contributor to obesity. Advances in technology, urbanization, and sedentary occupations have led to a decrease in physical activity levels. Many individuals spend a significant amount of time engaged in activities that involve minimal or no physical exertion such as watching television, playing video games, or browsing the internet. The lack of physical activity not only impedes caloric expenditure but also negatively impacts overall metabolic health.

Socioeconomic factors also play a significant role. People with lower income and education levels often face limited access to affordable, nutritious foods. They may reside in neighborhoods with limited or no supermarkets, commonly referred to as "food deserts." In these areas, fast-food restaurants and convenience stores offering unhealthy food choices are more readily available. Moreover, individuals with lower socioeconomic status may lack the resources and time to engage in regular physical activity or access to healthcare services.

Psychological factors, such as stress and emotional eating, contribute to the development of obesity. Stress can lead to an increase in the production of cortisol, a hormone that influences appetite and cravings for high-calorie foods. Individuals often turn to comfort foods as a coping mechanism, which can further contribute to weight gain. Moreover, psychological factors such as depression and low self-esteem can negatively impact lifestyle behaviors, leading to unhealthy dietary choices and sedentary habits.

Genetics and family history also play a significant role in obesity. Certain genetic variations can influence metabolism, appetite regulation, and the distribution of body fat. People with a family history of obesity are more likely to develop the condition themselves, suggesting a hereditary component. However, genetics alone cannot account for the drastic increase in obesity rates seen worldwide, indicating that environmental factors also play a crucial role.

Environmental factors encompass a range of influences, from the built environment to societal norms. The built environment refers to the physical infrastructure and resources available in a particular area. Neighborhoods with limited access to safe recreational spaces, sidewalks, or bike lanes can discourage physical activity. On the other hand, an environment that promotes physical activity, such as well-maintained parks and recreational facilities, can help combat obesity. Furthermore, societal norms and cultural influences surrounding food choices and portion sizes can significantly impact dietary behaviors.

Addressing the roots of obesity requires a multifaceted approach. Public health interventions aimed at promoting healthy eating habits and physical activity are key. This includes implementing policies to improve the nutritional quality of food options in schools, workplaces, and public spaces. Education and awareness campaigns can help individuals make informed choices about their diet and lifestyle. Additionally, creating environments that facilitate physical activity, such as creating walkable communities and promoting active transportation, is essential.

The roots of obesity are complex and multifactorial. Unhealthy diet, physical inactivity, socioeconomic factors, psychological influences, genetics, and environmental factors all play a significant role in the development of obesity. Tackling this global health issue requires a comprehensive approach that addresses these various factors. By promoting healthy lifestyles, improving access to nutritious foods, and creating supportive environments, we can work towards combating obesity and improving the overall health and well-being of individuals worldwide.

Obesity has become a global health epidemic, with rising rates affecting both developed and developing countries. It is a complex condition with numerous contributing factors, including genetic predisposition, environmental influences, individual behavior, and societal norms. Understanding the roots of obesity requires exploring these underlying factors, which interact in complex ways to influence an individual's likelihood of developing obesity.

One of the primary contributors to obesity is genetic predisposition. Research has demonstrated that genetics play a role in determining an individual's susceptibility to gaining weight. Certain genetic variations can affect metabolism, appetite regulation, and fat storage, making some individuals more susceptible to obesity than others.

However, it is important to note that genetics alone do not determine one's obesity status. Rather, they interact with other factors to influence weight gain.

Environmental influences also play a significant role in the development of obesity. With the ubiquity of high-calorie, processed foods, coupled with sedentary lifestyles, individuals have become more prone to weight gain. The availability and accessibility of unhealthy food options, such as fast food and sugary beverages, contribute to overeating and poor diet choices. Additionally, sedentary behaviors, including increased screen time and decreased physical activity, have become prevalent in modern society, further exacerbating the obesity crisis.

Individual behavior and lifestyle choices also contribute to the roots of obesity. Poor dietary choices, excessive calorie consumption, and lack of physical activity all contribute to weight gain. Factors such as emotional eating, stress, and lack of knowledge about nutrition also influence individual behavior. Additionally, cultural norms and societal expectations around body image can impact an individual's relationship with food and exercise. For instance, the emphasis on thinness in some societies can lead to disordered eating patterns, while the acceptance of larger body sizes in others may promote overeating and sedentary behavior.

Societal factors and policies also have a significant impact on obesity rates. The food industry's marketing practices, which often promote unhealthy food choices, contribute to the obesogenic environment. Furthermore, socioeconomic factors such as poverty and limited access to healthy foods, commonly referred to as food deserts, contribute to obesity disparities. Inequities in access to quality healthcare, education, and recreational facilities also contribute to the roots of obesity, as these factors can limit individuals' ability to engage in healthy behaviors and seek appropriate healthcare interventions.

Addressing the roots of obesity requires a multi-faceted approach that acknowledges the complexity of the issue. Firstly, education and awareness campaigns are crucial in promoting healthy eating habits, nutritional literacy, and the importance of physical activity. Providing accessible and affordable options for nutritious foods, especially in underserved communities, can help combat food insecurity and reduce reliance on unhealthy choices. Government policies and regulations that promote healthier food environments, such as imposing taxes on sugary beverages or implementing stricter marketing regulations, can also contribute to combating obesity.

Preventive efforts should also focus on inculcating healthier lifestyle habits from an early age. Schools can play a crucial role in promoting physical activity, providing balanced meals, and teaching children about nutrition. Creating supportive environments at home, work, and within the community that encourage healthy behaviors and discourage sedentary living is essential.

In conclusion, the roots of obesity are deeply intertwined with various factors, including genetic predisposition, environmental influences, individual behavior, and societal norms. Understanding these factors is essential in developing effective strategies to combat and prevent obesity. It requires a comprehensive approach involving education, policy changes, access to healthy foods, and creating supportive environments that promote healthy lifestyles. By addressing these roots, we can work towards a healthier future and reduce the burden of obesity globally.

CHAPTER 11: The hormonal causes and effects of overweight.

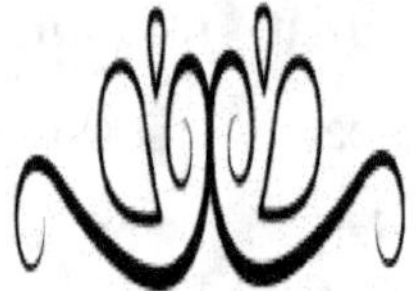

The hormonal causes and effects of obesity.

The hormonal causes and effects of obesity are complex and multifaceted, involving a delicate interplay between various hormones and physiological processes within the body. Obesity, defined as excessive accumulation of body fat, is influenced by both genetic and environmental factors, with hormonal imbalances playing a significant role in its development and progression.

One of the key hormones involved in the regulation of body weight is leptin. Leptin is produced by fat cells and acts as a satiety hormone, signaling the brain to reduce food intake and increase energy expenditure. In individuals with obesity, there is often a state of leptin resistance, where the body fails to respond appropriately to the hormone's signals. This resistance can lead to increased hunger, decreased satiety, and reduced energy expenditure, contributing to weight gain and difficulty in losing weight.

Another hormone involved in the regulation of body weight is ghrelin. Ghrelin is primarily produced in the stomach and stimulates appetite. Its levels increase before meals, signaling hunger to the brain. In individuals with obesity, there may be an imbalance in ghrelin regulation, leading to increased appetite and food cravings. This dysregulation can further contribute to overeating and weight gain.

Insulin, a hormone produced by the pancreas, plays a crucial role in regulating blood sugar levels. It helps facilitate the uptake of glucose into cells for energy production. However, in individuals with obesity, insulin resistance often develops, where cells become less responsive to the hormone's actions. This insulin resistance can lead to elevated insulin levels in the blood, promoting fat storage and inhibiting fat breakdown. It can also contribute to the development of type 2 diabetes, a condition often associated with obesity.

Additionally, adiponectin, a hormone secreted by fat cells, plays a role in regulating insulin sensitivity and inflammation. Lower levels of adiponectin are often observed in individuals with obesity, contributing to insulin resistance and increased risk of metabolic disorders. The hormonal imbalances associated with obesity can have a range of effects on various physiological processes. These effects can include:

1. **Increased appetite and food cravings:** Hormonal dysregulation can lead to heightened hunger signals and a

desire for calorie-dense foods, contributing to overeating and weight gain.

2. **Reduced satiety:** Leptin resistance can impair the brain's ability to recognize fullness, leading to a lack of satiety even after consuming adequate calories.

3. **Altered metabolism:** Hormonal imbalances can disrupt the body's metabolic rate, potentially leading to a slower metabolism and reduced energy expenditure.

4. **Fat storage:** Insulin resistance and elevated insulin levels promote fat storage, particularly in the abdominal region, increasing the risk of obesity-related health complications.

5. **Inflammation:** Adipose tissue, particularly visceral fat, releases inflammatory substances that can contribute to chronic low-grade inflammation, impairing metabolic function and increasing the risk of cardiovascular disease and other obesity-related conditions.

6. **Impaired glucose regulation:** Insulin resistance and dysregulated insulin levels can disrupt the body's ability to regulate blood sugar, increasing the risk of type 2 diabetes.

7. **Hormonal disruptions:** Obesity can disrupt the balance of various hormones involved in reproductive health, leading to menstrual irregularities, infertility, and hormonal imbalances.

8. **Cardiovascular complications:** Obesity-related hormonal imbalances, along with other factors like elevated cholesterol and blood pressure, can increase the risk of heart disease and stroke.

9. **Sleep disturbances:** Hormonal imbalances can contribute to sleep disorders such as sleep apnea, which are commonly associated with obesity.

10. **Psychological effects:** Hormonal imbalances and the societal stigma associated with obesity can contribute to psychological distress, including depression, anxiety, and low self-esteem.

It is important to note that the hormonal causes and effects of obesity can vary among individuals, and the interplay between hormones, genetics, and environmental factors is complex. Addressing hormonal imbalances in the context of obesity often requires a comprehensive approach that includes lifestyle modifications, dietary changes, physical activity, medication interventions, and, in some cases, bariatric surgery. Consulting with healthcare professionals, such as endocrinologists, registered dietitians, and psychologists, can provide personalized guidance and support in managing the hormonal aspects of obesity. Here is some information on the hormonal causes and effects of obesity, along with 10 tips, causes, functions, advantages, and disadvantages related to obesity.

Hormonal Causes and Effects of Obesity:

Obesity is a complex condition influenced by various hormonal factors. Hormones play a crucial role in regulating appetite, metabolism, and fat storage. Here are some key hormonal causes and effects of obesity:

1. **Leptin Resistance:** Leptin is a hormone that signals satiety to the brain. In obesity, the body becomes resistant to leptin, leading to decreased sensitivity to feelings of fullness.

2. **Insulin Resistance:** Insulin, known for its role in blood sugar regulation, also affects fat metabolism. Insulin resistance, often associated with obesity, reduces the body's ability to use insulin efficiently.

3. **Ghrelin Imbalance:** Ghrelin is a hormone that stimulates appetite. In obese individuals, ghrelin levels may be elevated, leading to increased hunger and overeating.

4. **Cortisol:** Chronic stress can elevate cortisol levels, which may contribute to weight gain and increased fat storage, particularly in the abdominal area.

5. **Sex Hormones:** Imbalances in sex hormones, such as estrogen and testosterone, can affect metabolism and fat distribution, potentially contributing to obesity.

6. **Thyroid Dysfunction:** An underactive thyroid (hypothyroidism) can lead to decreased metabolism, weight gain, and difficulty losing weight.

7. **Adiponectin Levels:** Adiponectin is a hormone that helps regulate glucose and fatty acid metabolism. Low levels of adiponectin are often found in obese individuals.

8. **Inflammatory Cytokines:** Inflammation plays a role in obesity. Increased production of inflammatory cytokines, such as TNF-alpha and IL-6, can contribute to insulin resistance and fat accumulation.

9. **Estrogen Dominance:** Excess estrogen relative to progesterone levels, often seen in conditions like polycystic

ovary syndrome (PCOS), can promote weight gain and fat storage.

10. **Genetic Factors:** Certain genetic predispositions can affect hormone regulation and contribute to obesity.

Tips for Managing Obesity:

1. Maintain a balanced and nutritious diet, rich in whole foods, fruits, vegetables, and lean proteins.
2. Engage in regular physical activity to promote calorie expenditure and improve metabolic rate.
3. Manage stress levels through techniques like meditation, deep breathing, or engaging in hobbies.
4. Get enough sleep to support hormonal regulation.
5. Avoid excessive consumption of processed and sugary foods that can disrupt hormonal balance.
6. Stay hydrated by drinking adequate amounts of water.
7. Gradually incorporate dietary changes rather than opting for crash diets.
8. Seek support from healthcare professionals, such as registered dietitians or therapists specializing in weight management.
9. Consider mindful eating practices, such as paying attention to hunger and fullness cues.
10. Be patient and maintain consistency, as sustainable weight loss takes time.

Causes of Obesity:

1. **Sedentary Lifestyle:** Lack of physical activity and prolonged periods of sitting or inactivity can contribute to weight gain.

2. **Poor Diet:** Overconsumption of calorie-dense, nutrient-poor foods, such as fast food and sugary beverages, is a leading cause of obesity.

3. **Genetic Factors:** Certain genetic variations can make individuals more prone to obesity.

4. **Environmental Factors:** Access to unhealthy food options, food marketing, and socioeconomic factors can contribute to obesity.

5. **Emotional Factors:** Emotional eating and using food as a coping mechanism can lead to weight gain.

6. **Medications:** Some medications, such as certain antidepressants or steroids, can contribute to weight gain.

7. **Lack of Sleep:** Sleep deprivation can disrupt hormonal regulation, leading to weight gain.

8. **Medical Conditions:** Certain medical conditions, such as hypothyroidism or PCOS, can contribute to obesity.

9. **Age:** Metabolism tends to slow down with age, making weight management more challenging.

10. **Socioeconomic Factors:** Limited access to affordable nutritious foods and opportunities for physical activity can contribute to obesity in lower-income communities.

Functions of Hormones in Obesity:

1. **Regulation of Appetite:** Hormones like leptin and ghrelin help regulate the sensation of hunger and fullness.

2. **Metabolic Rate Control:** Hormones, such as thyroid hormones and insulin, influence the body's metabolic rate and energy expenditure.

3. **Fat Storage Regulation:** Hormones like insulin and cortisol influence the storage and utilization of fat.

4. **Glucose Regulation:** Insulin plays a critical role in regulating blood sugar levels and preventing excessive glucose in the bloodstream.

5. **Inflammatory Response:** Hormones and inflammatory cytokines influence the body's inflammatory response, which can affect fat metabolism and insulin sensitivity.

6. **Lipid Metabolism:** Hormones like adiponectin play a role in regulating the breakdown and storage of fats.

7. **Hunger and Satiety Signaling:** Hormones like ghrelin and peptide YY (PYY) communicate hunger and satiety signals to the brain.

8. **Fat Distribution:** Hormones, including sex hormones, can influence how fat is distributed in the body.

9. **Insulin Sensitivity:** Hormones like insulin affect the body's sensitivity to the effects of insulin, which is important for blood sugar regulation.

10. **Hormone Interactions:** Hormones work together in a complex system, influencing and regulating each other's functions.

Advantages of Maintaining a Healthy Weight:

1. **Reduced Risk of Chronic Diseases:** Maintaining a healthy weight lowers the risk of conditions like heart disease, type 2 diabetes, and certain types of cancer.
2. **Improved Heart Health:** Being at a healthy weight helps lower blood pressure, reduce cholesterol levels, and improve overall cardiovascular function.
3. **Enhanced Mobility and Flexibility:** Carrying less weight reduces strain on joints and enhances physical mobility and flexibility.
4. **Increased Energy Levels:** Maintaining a healthy weight can lead to improved energy levels and overall vitality.
5. **Better Sleep Quality:** Achieving and maintaining a healthy weight can improve sleep quality and reduce the risk of sleep apnea.
6. **Improved Mental Well-being:** A healthy weight is associated with better mental health, increased self-esteem, and improved body image.
7. **Increased Fertility:** Obesity can impact fertility, and maintaining a healthy weight can improve reproductive health.
8. **Improved Digestive Health:** Maintaining a healthy weight can reduce the risk of gastrointestinal disorders and improve digestive function.

9. **Reduced Healthcare Costs:** Preventing obesity-related conditions can lead to reduced healthcare expenses in the long run.

10. **Enhanced Quality of Life:** Optimal weight management can improve overall quality of life, allowing for increased participation in activities and improved overall well-being.

Disadvantages of Obesity:

1. **Increased Risk of Chronic Diseases:** Obesity is associated with an increased risk of developing conditions such as heart disease, type 2 diabetes, stroke, and certain cancers.

2. **Reduced Mobility:** Obesity can limit physical mobility and make it more challenging to perform daily activities.

3. **Joint and Musculoskeletal Problems:** Excess weight puts additional strain on joints, leading to conditions like osteoarthritis.

4. **Sleep Apnea:** Obesity is a common risk factor for sleep apnea, a condition characterized by interruptions in breathing during sleep.

5. **Reduced Fertility:** Obesity can impair fertility and increase the risk of complications during pregnancy.

6. **Low Self-esteem and Body Image Issues:** Obesity can contribute to low self-esteem and body image dissatisfaction.

7. **Inflammation and Increased Risk of Infections:** Obesity is linked to chronic low-grade inflammation, which can weaken the immune system and increase the risk of infections.

8. **Mental Health Concerns:** Obesity is associated with an increased risk of mental health issues, such as depression and anxiety.

9. **Social Stigma:** Obese individuals may experience discrimination and social isolation, leading to negative psychosocial effects.

10. **Financial Burden:** Obesity can lead to increased healthcare costs, including medical treatments and managing obesity-related conditions.

Please note that this information is not exhaustive, and it is always recommended to consult healthcare professionals for personalized advice and treatment options related to obesity.

The hormonal causes and effects of obesity.

Numerous endocrine changes that result from modifications to the hypothalamic-pituitary hormone axis have been linked to obesity. These include hypogonadism, Cushing's illness, hypothyroidism, and a lack of growth hormone.

Hormones and obesity.

Hormones are chemical messengers that control bodily functions. They contribute to the development of obesity. Growth hormones, sex hormones, leptin, and insulin, as well as other hormones, have an impact on our body's metabolism (the rate at which it burns calories for energy), appetite, and body fat distribution. These hormones are present in higher amounts in obese people, which promotes an improper metabolism and the buildup of body fat. The endocrine system, a network of glands, secretes hormones into our bloodstream. The nervous system collaborates with the endocrine system and the immune system to aid our bodies in adjusting to various situations and challenges. Obesity can result from hormonal excesses or deficiencies, and vice versa; obesity can result from hormonal alterations.

Leptin and obesity.

Fat cells create the hormone leptin, which is then released into the bloodstream. By exerting its effects on particular brain regions, leptin lessens a person's desire to eat. It also appears to have a say in how the body handles its fat reserves. Leptin is created by fat, hence individuals who are obese typically have higher leptin levels than those who are of normal weight. However, despite having larger levels of this hormone that curbs appetite, obese persons are less sensitive to the effects of leptin and hence, tend to feel underestimated both during and after meals. The reason why leptin messages aren't reaching fat people's brains is still being investigated.

Insulin and obesity.

The pancreas secretes the hormone insulin, which is crucial for controlling carbohydrate and fat metabolism. Insulin encourages the blood's supply of glucose (sugar) to tissues like muscles, the liver, and fat. This procedure is crucial to maintaining appropriate levels of blood glucose and ensuring that there is energy available for daily activities. When insulin signals are lost in an obese person, tissues lose their ability to regulate glucose levels. This may result in the development of metabolic syndrome and type II diabetes.

Weight gain and sex hormones.

The distribution of body fat has a significant impact on the emergence of obesity-related illnesses such as heart disease, stroke, and various types of arthritis. A larger risk of disease is associated with abdominal fat than with fat that is stored on the hips, thighs, or bottom. It appears that androgens and estrogens influence how body fat is distributed. The ovaries in premenopausal women produce the sex hormones known as estrogens. They are in charge of starting ovulation at the beginning of each menstrual cycle. The testicles and ovaries of men and postmenopausal women do not produce a lot of estrogen. Instead, compared to what is created in pre-menopausal ovaries, the majority of their estrogen is made in body fat. Androgen production in the testes is high in younger males. These levels gradually decline as a guy ages. Variations in body fat distribution are related to changes in sex hormone levels with aging in both men and women. Older males and postmenopausal women tend to increase the storage of fat around their belly (making them more "apple-shaped"), whilst women of childbearing age tend to store fat in their lower body (making them more "pear-shaped"). Women who are postmenopausal and taking estrogen pills do not develop belly fat. Studies on animals have also demonstrated that a deficiency in estrogen causes excessive weight gain.

Growth hormone and obesity.

Growth hormone is produced by the pituitary gland in our brain, which affects a person's height and promotes the development of bone and muscle. Growth hormone influences metabolism as well (the rate at which we burn kilojoules for energy). Growth hormone levels have been discovered to be lower in obese individuals than in individuals of normal weight.

Obesity and inflammatory components.

Low-grade chronic inflammation within the fat tissue is another aspect of obesity. The release of pro-inflammatory substances from fat cells and immune cells within the adipose (fat) tissue is a result of stress reactions that occur within fat cells as a result of excessive fat buildup. The source of estrogen synthesis is crucial, as increased estrogen production in the fat of older obese women is linked to a higher risk of breast cancer.

Hormones linked to obesity and behavior.

Obese people have hormone levels that promote the buildup of body fat. Over time, it appears that habits like binge eating and skipping workouts 'reset' the mechanisms that control hunger and body fat distribution, making the person biologically more inclined to put on weight. The body fights against any temporary interruptions, like crash diets, because it is constantly attempting to preserve homeostasis. A low-calorie diet causes a person's blood leptin level to decrease, according to numerous studies. Lower levels of leptin may make someone more ravenous and their metabolism is slowed. This may help to explain why people who follow crash diets frequently put on the weight they lost. More study is required before leptin therapy becomes a reality, but it may one day assist dieters in long-term weight maintenance. The body may be re-trained to burn excess body fat and keep it off with long-term behavioral adjustments like a healthy diet and frequent exercise. Studies have also demonstrated that weight loss brought on by a balanced diet, regular exercise, or bariatric surgery improves insulin sensitivity, lowers inflammation, and advantageously modifies obesity hormones. Losing weight is also linked to a lower risk of heart disease, stroke, type II diabetes, and several types of cancer.

Obesity-Related To Endocrine Disorders.

Numerous endocrine changes that result from modifications to the hypothalamic-pituitary hormone axis have been linked to obesity. These include hypogonadism, Cushing's illness, hypothyroidism, and a lack of growth hormone. Adipocytes produce and release several hormones and chemicals, including leptin and adiponectin, which can mediate several other crucial functions of adipose tissue in addition to its involvement in energy storage. Hyperinsulinemia is the main etiological component of polycystic ovarian syndrome, which also frequently manifests as obesity.

How to Improve Your Hormones That Affect Your Weight.

Important chemicals that act as chemical messengers in your body are hormones. They support almost all physiological functions, such as metabolism, appetite, and fullness. Some hormones also play a crucial role in regulating hunger because of their connection to body mass. Here are the hormones that could have an impact on your weight, along with advice for maintaining appropriate levels of each.

1. Insulin.

Your pancreas produces insulin, which is the primary hormone used for storage in your body. Insulin encourages the storage of glucose, a simple sugar obtained from food, in the muscle, liver, and fat cells for later use in healthy humans. Small amounts of insulin are secreted throughout the day by your body, with greater amounts occurring after meals. Depending on your body's current needs, this hormone then transports glucose from food into your cells for either energy or storage. Your cells stop responding to insulin when you have insulin resistance, which is a fairly common condition. As a result of the insulin's inability to function, this condition causes high blood sugar glucosamine to enter your cells

Further insulin is subsequently produced by your pancreas to increase glucose absorption. Obesity has been linked to insulin resistance, which in turn may contribute to other illnesses like type 2 diabetes and heart disease. One can consider insulin sensitivity to be the polar opposite of insulin resistance. It indicates that your cells are insulin-sensitive. So it makes sense to concentrate on lifestyle practices that raise insulin sensitivity, such as the ones listed below.

Advice for increasing insulin sensitivity.

- Regular exercise. Exercise has been shown to increase insulin sensitivity and reduce insulin resistance when performed at high and moderate intensities.

- Change your sleeping patterns. Lack of sleep, particularly poor-quality sleep, is associated with insulin resistance and obesity.
- Up your intake of omega-3 fatty acids. According to research, omega-3 supplements may help persons with metabolic disorders like diabetes have better insulin sensitivity.
- If you dislike supplements, consider consuming more fish, nuts, seeds, and plant oils instead.
- Modify your diet. The Mediterranean diet, which is high in extra-virgin olive oil and healthful fats from nuts and seeds, may help lower insulin resistance. Reducing your consumption of saturated and trans fats may also be beneficial.
- Retain a healthy weight. Healthy weight loss and weight control may enhance insulin sensitivity in overweight individuals.
- Pay attention to low glycemic carbohydrates. Make the majority of your carbs low glycemic and high in fiber rather than trying to completely cut them out of your diet. Examples consist of whole grains, legumes, fruits, and veggies.

Chronic diseases including type 2 diabetes and heart disease are associated with insulin resistance. Focus on regular exercise, a nutritious diet, and improved sleeping patterns to increase insulin sensitivity.

2. Leptin.

Leptin is a hormone that promotes feeling full by signaling your hypothalamus, which controls your appetite, that you are full. Leptin resistance, however, may occur in obese people. This implies that the signal to quit eating doesn't get to your brain, ultimately leading to overeating. Your body may then continue to create more leptin until your levels rise. Leptin resistance may be caused by inflammation, gene mutations, or excessive leptin production, which can happen with obesity, although the exact cause is unknown.

hints for elevating leptin levels.

Leptin resistance has no known cure, however, several lifestyle adjustments may help reduce leptin levels.

- Keep a normal weight. It's crucial to keep a healthy weight because leptin resistance is linked to obesity. Furthermore, studies indicate that a reduction in body fat may assist in a reduction in leptin levels.
- Make your sleep better. In obese patients, leptin levels may be correlated with sleep quality. There are a lot of other reasons to get better sleep, even though this association might not be present in people who are not obese.
- Regular exercise. Leptin resistance, which prevents you from overeating, is found in obese people, and it has been linked in research to regular, consistent exercise.

According to research, regularly exercising, getting enough sleep, and Leptin levels can be decreased by exercising regularly and eating healthily.

3. Glutin.

Leptin and ghrelin are fundamentally antagonistic hormones. Your hypothalamus receives a signal from the hunger hormone telling it that your stomach is empty and that you need to eat. Its primary purpose is to improve hunger. Ghrelin levels are often highest before meals and lowest afterward. Curiously, studies show that obese individuals have lower ghrelin levels yet are more susceptible to its effects. This sensitivity could result in binge eating.

Advice on controlling ghrelin levels.

The fact that cutting calories frequently causes your ghrelin levels to rise and leave you feeling hungry is one reason why losing weight can be challenging. Additionally, leptin levels drop and metabolism tends to slow down. So, below are some suggestions for decreasing ghrelin to aid in appetite suppression:

- Keep a healthy body weight. Your sensitivity to ghrelin may grow as a result of obesity, which would therefore increase your hunger.
- Make an effort to sleep soundly. Increases in ghrelin, overeating, and weight gain can all result from lack of sleep.
- Consistently eat. Pre-meal ghrelin levels are at their peak, so pay attention to your body's cues and eat when you're hungry.

The effects of the hunger hormone ghrelin may be felt more keenly by obese people. According to research, controlling this hormone is aided by keeping a healthy body weight and giving sleep priority.

4. Cortisol.

Your adrenal glands create cortisol, sometimes known as the stress hormone. This hormone causes an increase in energy and heart rate when under stress. Cortisol is released together with the frequently referred to as the "fight or flight" reaction, the hormone adrenaline While your body must release cortisol in dangerous circumstances, prolonged high amounts can cause several health problems, such as diabetes, heart disease, low energy, high blood pressure, sleep disorders, and weight gain. High cortisol levels may be caused by several lifestyle choices, such as insufficient sleep, ongoing stress, and eating a lot of high-glycemic meals. Additionally, excessive levels of cortisol may lead to weight increase in addition to obesity, producing a negative feedback loop.

Suggestions for reducing cortisol.

The following lifestyle modifications could help control cortisol levels:

- Improve sleep. High blood pressure may be exacerbated by long-term sleep problems like insomnia, sleep apnea, and irregular sleeping patterns (like those of shift workers) cortisol amounts. Develop a consistent bedtime and sleep pattern.

- Regular exercise. High-intensity exercise briefly raises cortisol levels, while routine exercise often lowers levels by enhancing general health and reducing stress.
- Engage in mindfulness. There needs to be more research, however, it appears that mindfulness practice frequently lowers cortisol levels. Make meditation a part of your everyday practice.
- Keep a healthy body weight. Maintaining a moderate weight may assist keep levels in line because obesity may raise cortisol levels and excessive cortisol levels can lead to weight gain (37Trusted Source).
- Consume a healthy diet. According to research, diets high in refined grains, added sugars, and saturated fat may cause cortisol levels to rise. The Mediterranean diet may also assist in lowering cortisol levels.

Although cortisol is a critical hormone, persistently excessive amounts can cause diseases like diabetes, heart disease, and obesity. Your levels may be lowered by maintaining a nutritious diet, exercising frequently, getting enough sleep, and engaging in mindfulness exercises.

5. Estrogen.

Estrogen is a sex hormone that controls the immunological, skeletal, and circulatory systems in addition to the female reproductive system. The menstrual cycle and other life phases, including pregnancy, lactation, and menopause, affect hormone levels. High estrogen levels, which are frequently found in obese individuals, are linked to an increased risk of some malignancies and other chronic disorders. Conversely, low levels, which are frequently associated with aging, perimenopause, and menopause, may have an impact on body weight and body fat, raising your risk of chronic illnesses, Low estrogen levels frequently result in central obesity, which is a buildup of weight around the body's trunk. Other health issues like excessive blood sugar, high blood pressure, and heart disease may result from this. By making lifestyle adjustments, especially by keeping a healthy body weight, you can reduce your risk of developing many of these health problems.

Guidelines for maintaining normal estrogen levels.

Try some of these methods to maintain appropriate levels of estrogen:

- Work on controlling your weight. Due to low estrogen levels in women between the ages of 55 and 75, weight loss or maintenance may lower the risk of heart disease. Research also suggests maintaining a healthy weight to lower your risk of chronic diseases in general.

- Regular exercise. low amounts of estrogen may make you believe that you are less capable of exercising. Nevertheless, regular exercise is still essential to help with weight management during times of low estrogen secretion, such as menopause.

- Consume a healthy diet. It has been demonstrated that diets high in red meat, processed foods, sweets, and refined grains enhance estrogen levels, which may increase your chance of developing chronic diseases. As a result, you might want to restrict how often you eat these items.

- Your risk of disease may increase with both high and low levels of the sex hormone estrogen, so it's critical to maintain a healthy lifestyle to minimize these risks.

6. Norepinephrine Y.

Your brain and nerve system create a hormone called neuropeptide Y (NPY) that stimulates In reaction to stress or fasting, appetite falls and energy expenditure decreases. NPY is linked to obesity and weight gain because it may boost food consumption. It is activated in fat tissue, where it may increase fat storage, cause abdominal obesity, and result in metabolic syndrome, which raises the chance of developing chronic diseases. Research has demonstrated that the mechanisms through which NPY causes obesity may also result in an inflammatory reaction, further deteriorating health problems.

Guidelines for preserving low NPY levels

Here are some pointers for preserving normal levels of NPY:

- Workout. There is conflicting evidence, but some studies point to the possibility that regular exercise may help lower NPY levels.
- Consume a balanced diet. High-fat, high-sugar diets may raise NPY levels, though more research is needed in this area, so you might want to Reduce your consumption of foods that are heavy in sugar and fat.

- NPY is a hormone that increases appetite and has been linked to obesity. Regular exercise and a good diet could be beneficial for maintaining healthy levels. Receive no-cost, quick snack recipes.
- Let the dietitians at Healthline make suggestions for munchies based on your dietary needs and culinary preferences.

7. The peptide glucagon.

A hormone called glucagon-like peptide-1 (GLP-1) is created in the gut when food enters the intestines. It is crucial for stabilizing blood sugar levels and promoting satiety. According to research, obesity may cause issues with GLP-1 signaling. As a result, GLP-1 is included in pharmaceuticals, especially for those with diabetes, to help patients lose weight and shrink their waist circumference.

Tips for maintaining GLP-1 levels in control.

Here are some pointers to keep GLP-1 levels in a safe range:

- Consume a lot of protein. Yogurt and other high-protein foods, such as whey protein, have been demonstrated to raise GLP-1 levels.
- Think about consuming probiotics. Probiotics may raise GLP-1 levels, according to a preliminary study, but more human studies are required.
- Additionally, before beginning any new supplements, it's essential to speak with a healthcare expert.

GLP-1 is a hormone that causes fullness, although obese persons may not be as susceptible to its effects. Try to eat a well-rounded diet with lots of protein to keep your GLP-1 levels in check.

8. Cholecystokinin.

Cholecystokinin (CCK), like GLP-1, is a hormone that your gut produces after a meal to make you feel full. It is crucial for digestion, protein synthesis, energy production, and other physical processes. Leptin, a hormone that signals fullness, is also released more frequently. People who are obese may be less sensitive to the effects of CCK, which could result in chronic overeating. This could lead to a negative feedback loop by further lowering CCK sensitivity.

Guidelines for raising CCK levels

Here are some pointers for keeping CCK levels in a healthy range:

- Consume a lot of protein. According to certain studies, a high-protein diet may help raise CCK levels and, as a result, make you feel fuller.
- Workout. Despite the paucity of data, some evidence suggests that regular exercise can raise CCK levels.
- People with obesity may develop desensitization to the fullness hormone CCK. This could result in overeating. For a diet high in protein and regular exercise to keep CCK levels in check.

9. YY Peptide.

Another gut hormone that suppresses appetite is peptide PYY levels may be reduced in obese individuals, which may cause an increase in hunger and overeating. It is thought that adequate levels greatly contribute to lowering food consumption and lowering the risk of obesity.

How to increase PYY levels.

Here are some strategies for maintaining a healthy level of PYY in your body:

- **Consume a balanced diet.** Protein consumption in large amounts may support normal PYY levels and satiety. Furthermore, the paleo diet, which is high in protein, fruits, and vegetables, may cause PYY levels to increase, although further research is required.
- **Workout.** Although there is conflicting evidence, being active is typically good for health.
- **Obese individuals may have a low PYY level, which indicates fullness.** A high-protein diet and regular exercise may assist to increase levels.

CHAPTER 12: The Impact of Carbohydrates on Physical Appearance.

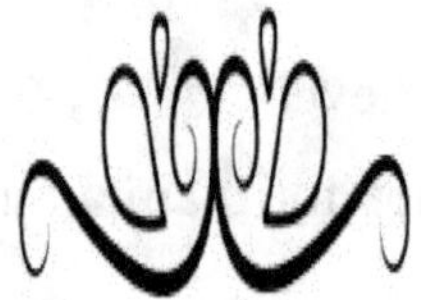

The Impact of Carbohydrates on Physical Appearance.

A Comprehensive Analysis.

Carbohydrates are an essential component of our diet, providing the body with energy and fulfilling various metabolic functions. However, there has been ongoing speculation about the influence of carbohydrates on physical appearance. This essay aims to delve into the scientific understanding of how carbohydrates impact our looks, considering factors such as weight management, muscle definition, and skin health.

Body:

I. Carbohydrates and Weight Management:

- A. Role of carbohydrates in energy production and storage.
- B. Understanding the glycemic index and its relationship to weight gain.

- C. Differentiating between complex and simple carbohydrates.
- D. Discussing the impact of carbohydrate consumption on body weight.

II. Carbohydrates and Muscle Definition:

- A. The role of carbohydrates in providing energy for exercise.
- B. Examining the correlation between carbohydrate intake and muscle glycogen stores.
- C. The importance of timing carbohydrate consumption for optimal muscle growth and recovery.
- D. Considering the protein-carbohydrate balance for muscle definition.

III. Carbohydrates and Skin Health:

- A. The link between high-glycemic carbohydrate consumption and skin conditions.
- B. Discussing how insulin levels affect the production of androgens and sebum.
- C. Examining the impact of carbohydrate-rich diets on acne and aging.
- D. Highlighting the benefits of low-glycemic carbohydrates for maintaining healthy skin

IV. Carbohydrate Quality and Overall Physical Appearance:

- A. Focusing on whole grains, fruits, and vegetables as healthier carbohydrate sources.
- B. The role of dietary fiber in promoting satiety and weight management.
- C. Discussing the impact of refined and processed carbohydrates on body composition.
- D. Emphasizing the importance of a balanced diet for overall physical appearance

Conclusion:

In conclusion, carbohydrates do have an impact on how we look, but this impact is multifaceted and depends on various factors. While excessive consumption of refined carbohydrates may contribute to weight gain and skin issues, moderate intake of complex carbohydrates, such as fruits, vegetables, and whole grains, can aid in weight management, muscle definition, and skin health. It is crucial to consider the quality and quantity of carbohydrate consumption as part of a balanced diet, alongside other lifestyle factors, to achieve and maintain a desired physical appearance. Therefore, understanding and making informed choices about carbohydrates can positively influence our overall looks and well-being.

CHAPTER 13: Enrichment and upgrading of flour.

Enrichment and upgrading of flour.

Enrichment and upgrading of flour refer to the process of enhancing the nutritional content, quality, and functionality of flour. Flour is a fundamental ingredient in many food products, and by enriching and upgrading it, manufacturers can improve the nutritional value and overall performance of their food products. This article will provide a summary of the enrichment and upgrading techniques used in flour processing.

Flour is primarily made from grinding grains such as wheat, corn, or rice. It is commonly used in bread, pastries, pasta, and various other food products. However, the milling process used to produce flour often removes certain parts of the grain, including the bran and germ, which contain many valuable nutrients. As a result, the flour obtained from this process is often nutritionally deficient.

To address this issue, flour enrichment was introduced. Enriched flour is produced by adding back certain nutrients that are lost during milling. The most common nutrients added to enriched flour include iron, thiamin (vitamin B1), riboflavin (vitamin B2), niacin (vitamin B3), and folic acid (vitamin B9). These nutrients are essential for human health and play a crucial role in various bodily functions.

The enrichment process involves carefully measuring and adding the required amounts of nutrients to the flour. This is typically done in large-scale flour mills or food processing facilities. By enriching the flour, manufacturers aim to compensate for the nutrient loss that occurs during milling, ensuring that the final product provides a certain level of essential nutrients.

In addition to enrichment, flour can also be upgraded through various techniques to improve its quality and functionality. These techniques include fortification, blending, and customization.

Fortification involves adding additional nutrients to flour beyond what is typically found in enriched flour. This can include adding vitamins such as vitamin D or vitamin E, minerals like calcium or zinc, or other beneficial substances like fiber or omega-3 fatty acids. Fortified flour is often used to address specific nutritional deficiencies or to meet the dietary needs of specific populations, such as pregnant women or children.

Blending is another technique used to upgrade flour. It involves combining different types of flours to create a product with specific characteristics. For example, blending wheat flour with legume flours like chickpea or lentil flour can increase the protein content and improve the amino acid profile of the final product. Blending can also be used to enhance the taste, texture, or color of flour-based foods.

Customization refers to tailoring the flour characteristics to meet specific requirements. This can involve modifying the particle size, moisture content, or gluten content of the flour. Customized flour is often used in industrial food production where specific flour properties are needed for optimal processing and product quality.

In recent years, advancements in food science and technology have enabled the development of innovative flour upgrading techniques. For example, micronization is a process that involves grinding flour into very fine particles, enhancing its functional properties, such as improved water absorption and dough stability. Another technique called extrusion can be used to modify the starch structure in flour, resulting in improved texture, flavor, and digestibility.

The enrichment and upgrading of flour have significant benefits for both consumers and food manufacturers. For consumers, enriched and upgraded flour products offer improved nutritional value, ensuring the intake of essential nutrients. These products can also provide enhanced taste, texture, and overall quality, making them more appealing to consumers.

For food manufacturers, using enriched and upgraded flour can enhance the nutritional profile and marketability of their products. It allows them to meet the growing demand for healthier and more nutritious food options. Additionally, upgrading flour can improve the functionality of the flour, making it easier to work with in various food processing applications.

In conclusion, the enrichment and upgrading of flour involve techniques aimed at improving the nutritional content, quality, and functionality of flour. Enrichment involves adding back essential nutrients lost during milling, while upgrading techniques such as fortification, blending, and customization enhance the nutritional profile and functional properties of flour. These processes have significant benefits for both consumers and food manufacturers, ensuring the availability of healthier and more nutritious food options in the market.

Enrichment and upgrading of flour is a process that involves enhancing the nutritional content and quality of flour through various methods. Here are some details regarding tips, causes, functions, advantages, and disadvantages related to this process:

Tips for Enrichment and Upgrading of Flour:

1. **Use fortified flour:** Look for flour that is specifically labeled as enriched or fortified to ensure higher nutritional value.
2. **Opt for whole-grain flour:** Whole-grain flour contains more nutrients than refined flour, making it a healthier choice.

3. **Check the expiration date:** Ensure that the flour you purchase is fresh to maintain its nutrient content.

4. **Store flour properly:** Store flour in a cool, dry place to prevent nutrient degradation.

5. **Consider organic options:** Organic flour is often produced without the use of synthetic chemicals, making it a more natural choice.

6. **Experiment with alternative flours:** Experiment with different types of flour to diversify your nutrient intake.

7. **Combine different flours:** Mixing various types of flour can result in a more balanced nutritional profile.

8. **Pay attention to processing methods:** Choose flours that are minimally processed to preserve more nutrients.

9. **Learn about baking techniques:** Understand the effects of different flours on baking to make the best use of their nutritional benefits.

10. **Read labels carefully:** Familiarize yourself with the ingredients and nutritional information provided on flour packaging.

Causes of Enrichment and Upgrading of Flour:

1. **Nutritional deficiencies:** Flour enrichment is carried out to address deficiencies common in certain populations.

2. **Improving public health:** Fortifying flour with additional nutrients can help combat widespread nutrient deficiencies and promote better health.

3. **Regulatory requirements:** Some countries have regulations that mandate the fortification of certain staple foods, including flour.
4. **Enhancing consumer choices:** Offering a wider range of nutritionally fortified flours allows consumers to make healthier choices.
5. **Addressing specific dietary needs:** Enriched flour can cater to the needs of individuals who require additional nutrients in their diet.
6. **Supporting child development:** Fortifying flour with key nutrients like iron and B vitamins helps in the healthy growth and development of children.
7. **Tackling malnutrition:** Upgrading flour can be an important strategy for reducing malnutrition in communities.
8. **Combating food insecurity:** Fortified flour can contribute to improving the availability and nutritional quality of staple foods.
9. **Reducing micronutrient deficiencies:** Enrichment addresses the lack of essential vitamins and minerals in diets that can lead to deficiencies.
10. **Promoting overall well-being:** Enhancing the nutritional value of flour contributes to better overall health and vitality.

Functions of Enriched and Upgraded Flour:

1. **Nutrient supplementation:** The primary function of enriched flour is to provide additional nutrients that may be lacking in the diet.

2. **Preventing deficiencies:** Fortified flour helps prevent nutrient deficiencies that can have detrimental effects on health.

3. **Enhancing the nutritional profile:** Upgrading flour increases its content of essential vitamins and minerals, improving its overall nutritional value.

4. **Supporting energy production:** Enriched flour provides vital nutrients that are involved in energy metabolism.

5. **Strengthening the immune system**: Fortified flour can contain vitamins and minerals that play a role in maintaining a robust immune system.

6. **Supporting cognitive function:** Certain nutrients in enriched flour, such as B vitamins, are essential for maintaining healthy brain function.

7. **Promoting healthy digestion:** Some flours can be fortified with dietary fiber, which aids in digestion and promotes gut health.

8. **Contributing to healthy growth and development:** Fortified flour provides key nutrients needed for proper growth and development in children and adolescents.

9. **Enhancing food taste and texture:** Upgraded flour can improve the quality, taste, and texture of baked goods.

10. **Facilitating food preservation:** Certain fortification methods can enhance the shelf life and stability of flour products.

Advantages of Enrichment and Upgrading of Flour:

1. **Improved nutrient intake:** Enriched flour offers a convenient way to ensure adequate intake of essential nutrients.

2. **Addressing nutritional gaps:** Fortifying flour helps bridge the gap between nutrient requirements and actual dietary intake.

3. **Public health benefits:** Enrichment programs can contribute to reducing the prevalence of nutrient deficiencies in populations.

4. **Cost-effectiveness:** Fortification is often a cost-effective strategy for improving public health outcomes compared to individual supplementation.

5. **Wide accessibility:** Enriched flour is widely available, making it accessible to a large population and promoting equitable access to nutrients.

6. **Contribution to food security:** Fortified flour can enhance the nutrient content of staple foods, addressing food security challenges in vulnerable populations.

7. **Flexibility in consumption:** Upgraded flour can be easily incorporated into various recipes and food preparations, providing flexibility in consumption patterns.

8. **Ease of implementation:** The process of enriching and upgrading flour is technologically feasible and can be seamlessly integrated into existing production methods.

9. **Positive impact on specific populations:** Fortifying flour can have particular benefits for high-risk groups such as pregnant women, children, and the elderly.

10. **Collaboration between various sectors:** Enrichment initiatives often involve collaborations between governments, food manufacturers, and public health agencies, fostering multi-sector partnerships.

Disadvantages of Enrichment and Upgrading of Flour:

1. **Loss of natural nutrients:** The process of upgrading flour can result in the loss of certain natural nutrients during milling and fortification.

2. **Limited nutrient range:** Fortification targets specific nutrients, potentially leaving out other essential compounds found naturally in whole foods.

3. **Potential for overconsumption:** Relying solely on enriched flour may lead to overconsumption of certain nutrients if other dietary sources are not diversified.

4. **Risk of nutrient imbalances:** Over-reliance on fortified flour without a balanced diet may lead to imbalances in nutrient intake.

5. **Bioavailability concerns:** The bioavailability of certain fortified nutrients may vary, affecting their absorption and utilization by the body.

6. **Cost implications:** Fortified flour can be more expensive than regular flour, potentially posing affordability challenges for low-income individuals.

7. **Technological limitations:** Some nutrients may be difficult to incorporate into flour due to stability and processing constraints.
8. **Potential for sensory changes:** Fortification may alter the taste, color, or texture of flour, potentially impacting consumer acceptance.
9. **Regulatory challenges:** Implementing and ensuring compliance with fortification regulations can pose administrative and enforcement challenges.
10. **Lack of awareness and education:** Consumer awareness about the benefits and appropriate use of fortified flour may be limited, hindering its impact on public health.

It's important to note that specific advantages and disadvantages may vary based on regional regulations, fortification methods, and individual dietary needs.

CHAPTER 14: Sugar Role in Making You Fat.

Sugar Role in Making You Fat.

Sugar consumption has been a major concern for public health due to its association with weight gain and obesity. In this article, we will explore the effects of sugar on body weight and outline its role in making you fat. Additionally, we will discuss 10 tips to reduce sugar intake, 10 causes of excessive sugar consumption, 10 factors contributing to weight gain, 10 benefits of reducing sugar intake, as well as 10 advantages and disadvantages of sugar consumption.

Sugar is a type of carbohydrate commonly found in processed foods, beverages, and sweets. It provides a quick source of energy but can be detrimental when consumed excessively. High sugar consumption can lead to weight gain and obesity due to various reasons.

Firstly, sugar is calorie-dense. It provides empty calories without essential nutrients, which can result in an imbalance between calorie intake and expenditure. When consumed in excess, the body stores the unused calories as fat, leading to weight gain over time.

Secondly, consuming sugary foods and beverages can lead to overeating. Sugar triggers the pleasure centers in the brain, causing cravings and addiction-like behaviors. This can result in a higher calorie intake, potentially leading to weight gain if not balanced with physical activity.

Thirdly, sugar-sweetened beverages like sodas and fruit juices can be particularly harmful. These drinks often contain a high amount of sugar and do not provide the same sensation of fullness as solid foods. As a result, people tend to consume more calories overall when regularly consuming sugary beverages.

Tips.

Let's explore few tips to reduce sugar intake:

1. **Read food labels:** Be mindful of hidden sugars in processed foods and choose options with low sugar content.
2. **Avoid sugary drinks:** Opt for water, herbal tea, or unsweetened beverages instead of soda or fruit juice.
3. **Be cautious with condiments:** Sauces and dressings can contain hidden sugars, so choose low-sugar alternatives or make your own.
4. **Choose whole foods:** Focus on consuming whole fruits, vegetables, and unprocessed foods that have naturally occurring sugars.

5. **Cook at home:** By preparing meals at home, you have better control over the ingredients and can reduce sugar content.

6. **Limit processed snacks:** Processed snacks like cookies, cakes, and candies are often high in added sugars. Choose healthier alternatives like nuts, seeds, or homemade snacks.

7. **Be mindful of sugar substitutes:** Artificial sweeteners may have fewer calories, but they can still trigger cravings and contribute to overeating. Moderation is key.

8. **Establish a meal routine:** Having regular, balanced meals can help prevent excessive sugar cravings and overeating.

9. **Practice stress management:** Emotional eating is often associated with sugary foods. Find healthier ways to cope with stress, such as exercise, meditation, or hobbies.

10. **Seek support:** Share your goals with friends or join a support group to stay motivated and accountable when reducing sugar intake.

Causes.

Let's explore some causes of excessive sugar consumption:

1. **Marketing and advertising:** The food industry heavily promotes sugary foods, making them easily accessible and appealing.

2. **Convenience and availability:** Processed foods and sugary beverages are readily available and often more convenient than healthier options.

3. **Emotional eating:** Many people turn to sugary foods as a way to cope with stress, sadness, or boredom.

4. **Lack of nutrition education:** Some individuals may not be aware of the negative effects of excessive sugar consumption or lack knowledge about healthier alternatives.

5. **Cultural and societal norms:** Certain cultures or social settings may prioritize or associate sugary foods with celebrations or social gatherings.

6. **Lack of time for meal preparation:** Busy schedules may lead to a reliance on processed foods or takeout, which often contain higher sugar content.

7. **Taste preferences:** Sweet tastes are naturally appealing, and the food industry often capitalizes on this by adding excess sugar to products.

8. **Food addiction:** Sugar can be addictive, causing individuals to crave and rely on sugary foods.

9. **Psychological factors:** Some individuals may have a predisposition to overeating or have emotional attachments to sugary foods.

10. **Lack of wise food choices:** Simply not prioritizing nutritious and low-sugar foods can contribute to excessive sugar consumption.

Factors.

Let's discuss few factors contributing to weight gain:

1. **High sugar intake:** Excessive sugar consumption contributes to excess calorie intake and fat storage.

2. **Sedentary lifestyle:** Lack of physical activity leads to fewer calories burned, making it easier to gain weight.

3. **Poor dietary choices:** Consuming high-calorie, low-nutrient foods contributes to weight gain.

4. **Portion sizes:** Oversized portions can lead to calorie excess, resulting in weight gain.

5. **Stress and emotional eating:** Using food as a coping mechanism for stress or emotions can lead to weight gain.

6. **Lack of sleep:** Sleep deprivation can disrupt hormonal balance, leading to increased appetite and weight gain.

7. **Genetics:** Some individuals may have genetic predispositions that make it more challenging to maintain a healthy weight.

8. **Medications:** Certain medications may have side effects that contribute to weight gain.

9. **Hormonal changes:** Hormonal imbalances can affect metabolism and promote weight gain.

10. **Aging:** As we age, our metabolism naturally slows down, increasing the likelihood of weight gain.

Benefits.

Let's explore some benefits of reducing sugar intake:

1. **Weight management:** Reducing sugar intake can help maintain a healthy body weight and prevent weight gain.

2. **Improved energy levels:** Consuming less sugar reduces blood sugar fluctuations, leading to more stable energy levels throughout the day.

3. **Reduced risk of type 2 diabetes:** Excessive sugar consumption is closely linked to the development of type 2 diabetes. Limiting sugar intake may help prevent or manage the condition.

4. **Better dental health:** High sugar intake is a major contributor to tooth decay. Reducing sugar consumption can improve oral health.

5. **Reduced inflammation:** Excess sugar can promote inflammation in the body. Cutting back on sugar may help decrease inflammation and associated health risks.

6. **Lower risk of heart disease:** Excessive sugar intake is associated with heart disease risk factors such as obesity, high blood pressure, and high cholesterol levels. Reducing sugar consumption can improve heart health.

7. **Enhanced brain function:** A high-sugar diet has been linked to cognitive decline. By reducing sugar intake, brain health and cognitive function can be improved.

8. **Balanced mood:** Sugar crashes and blood sugar fluctuations can affect mood stability. Cutting back on sugar can promote more stable moods.

9. **Improved skin health:** High sugar intake can contribute to skin issues like acne and premature aging. Reducing sugar may lead to better skin health.

10. **Overall improved nutrition:** Choosing low-sugar options encourages the consumption of nutrient-dense foods, leading to improved overall nutrition.

Let's discuss few advantages and disadvantages of sugar consumption.

Advantages:

1. Quick source of energy.
2. Enhances taste and flavor in food.
3. Provides some essential nutrients in natural forms like fruits.
4. Boosts serotonin levels, potentially improving mood temporarily.
5. Can be used as a fuel source during endurance activities.

Disadvantages:

1. Empty calories without essential nutrients.
2. Contributes to weight gain and obesity.
3. Increases the risk of chronic diseases like diabetes and heart disease.
4. May promote inflammation in the body.
5. Can lead to dental issues like tooth decay.

In summary, excessive sugar consumption plays a significant role in weight gain and obesity. To reduce sugar intake, follow the 10 tips mentioned earlier, while being aware of the 10 causes and factors that contribute to weight gain. Reducing sugar intake offers numerous benefits, including weight management, improved energy levels, reduced risk of diseases, and better overall health. However, it is essential to recognize that sugar consumption does have some advantages, but the disadvantages outweigh them when consumed in excess. Prioritizing a balanced and moderate approach to sugar consumption is crucial for maintaining optimal health and preventing weight gain.

www.ingramcontent.com/pod-product-compliance
Lightning Source LLC
Chambersburg PA
CBHW070936260726
48661CB00003B/1013